# Hormone Therapies In Chronic Pain Care



Forest Tennant, DrPH, MPH, MD

ISBN: 9781955934510
Library of Congress Control Number: 2026903164

Special discounts are available on quantity purchases by corporations, associations, educators, and others. For details, contact one of the parties listed below.

U.S. trade bookstores and wholesalers: Please contact Nancy Kriskovich Tel: (406)249-2002;
or email snkriskovich@gmail.com

All proceeds from the sale of this book will go to Arachnoiditis Hope sponsored by the
Tennant Foundation
336-338 S. Glendora Ave.
West Covina, CA 91790-3043
Ph: 626-716-2689
Fax: 626-919-7497
Email: tennantfoundation92@gmail.com

Published by the
Tennant Foundation
West Covina, California

SPONSORS OF THIS BOOK
Tennant Foundation
336-338 S. Glendora Ave.
West Covina, CA 91790-3043
Ph: 626-716-2689
Fax: 626-919-7497
Email: tennantfoundation92@gmail.com

## Publication Development

Rebecca Cholcher-Marino
Nancy Kriskovich

## Advisory Board

Judy Beaver, RN
Andrew Boyles
Donna Corley
Scott Guess, PharmD
Alison Guyton
Ryle Holder, PharmD
Ingrid Hollis
Sarah Lewis
Carol Mathews, RN, NP
Kristen Ogden
Jaime Sanchez, RN
Michael Seidel
Julie Utz

# DEDICATION

To my wife, Miriam, who throughout 60 years of marriage has supported and encouraged me every step of the way.

# Contents

# Author's Notes

I have written this book because I strongly believe it is time to incorporate hormonal therapies into the care of essentially every chronic pain patient. Despite an imperfect chronic pain care system that admittedly has some supply, regulation, and financial issues, modern chronic pain management has achieved great success. Recently developed medications, physical therapies, and surgical procedures have brought humanitarian relief and recovery to millions around the world. Some hormones can and will build on this foundation.

Hormones enhance chronic pain care by either potentiating analgesia and/or by treating the underlying cause of pain. I have done a number of studies on hormones in pain care and administered hormones for various purposes to countless chronic pain patients. There is a plethora of basic science studies involving hormones in pain care. In this book, I've attempted to combine my experiences with these studies. I have written this book in the hope that every chronic pain patient and medical practitioner can find at least one clinical tip or pearl to enhance their care of chronic pain. I've attached a "quick clinical guide" with some hormones to help practitioners pick and choose hormone therapies that fit their practice. Modern pain treatment has made considerable advances. Millions of persons have benefitted from new therapeutic measures and medicinals. Hormones are the "new kid on the block," and one that will move chronic pain care a step forward.

# 1. Introduction

The main intent of this book is to assist patients and practitioners identify hormonal therapies that will enhance or embellish their current medical treatment regimen. Hormones are not a substitute for today's menu of pharmacologic and non-pharmacologic treatments, but therapeutic measures to treat the underlying cause of pain and enhance pain relief medications.

Hormones are substances that originate in a gland or other body part that is conveyed in the blood to other body parts to stimulate some physiological function. Some hormones will reduce pain, potentiate analgesic agents, and/or treat the underlying cause of pain. Various hormones suppress inflammation and autoimmunity, regenerate or heal damaged tissues, and/or activate neurotransmitter-receptor systems in the central nervous system (CNS). This book describes how to use hormones to enhance chronic pain care.

TABLE

## Major Pain Control Mechanisms of Hormones

### Pain-Control Mechanisms

- Anti-inflammatory action
- Cellular metabolism
- Cellular protection
- Glucose control
- Immunoreactivity
- Tissue regeneration

### Central Nervous System Functions

- Receptor binding
- Nerve conduction
- Maintenance of blood-brain barrier

| Today's Major Causes of Severe Chronic Pain |
| --- |
| Adhesive Arachnoiditis |
| Chronic Regional Pain Syndrome (CRPS) |
| Ehlers-Danlos Syndrome |
| Cervical Neuropathy |
| Bone on bone arthritis |
| Multi-system disease* |
| Fibromyalgia |
| Irritable bowel |
| Migraine |
| Small fiber neuropathy |
| Pudendal Neuropathy |

Today's Major Causes of Severe Chronic Pain

*Today a high percentage of chronic pain patients have multiple pain conditions (i.e., fibromyalgia, herniated discs, arthritis, irritable bowel, migraine, etc.) which may have one or more underlying causes.

TABLE

The Hormonal Pathway in Adrenals, Gonads, and Central Nervous System

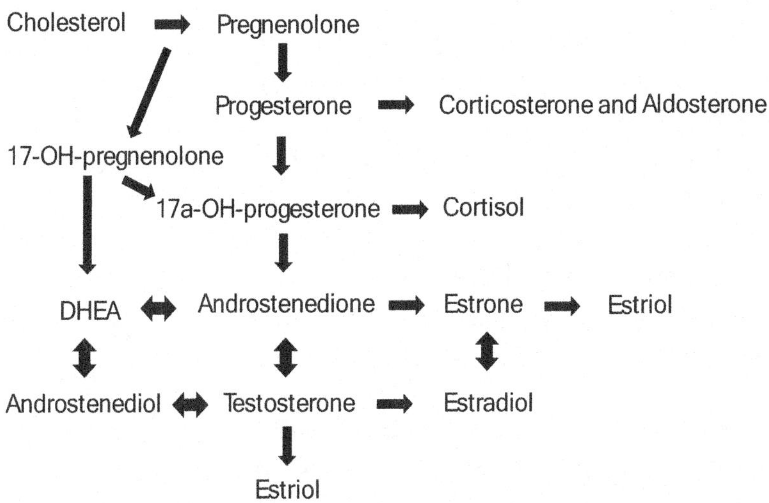


Note that pregnenolone is the base or precursor hormone for all other hormones. Also note that DHEA metabolizes to testosterone and estradiol. The above hormonal pathway is operable in the adrenals, gonads, and central nervous system.

# 2. HORMONE DEFICIENCIES: CONSTANT ISSUE

Hormonal deficiencies are a constant occurrence in chronic pain patients. Unfortunately, both chronic pain and the medicinals used to treat it can suppress some hormone production. A basic therapeutic measure in pain care is to determine the blood level of hormones that are deficient and then replace them. Physiologically, pain is a severe stress state that stimulates the hypothalamus and pituitary gland to produce extra levels of adrenocorticotrophin hormone (ACTH), follicle stimulating hormone (FSH), and luteinizing hormone (LH), which are the hormones that stimulate the adrenal glands, ovaries, and testicles to produce key hormones such as cortisol, estrogen, and testosterone.

Unfortunately, uncontrolled pain can overstress the pituitary gland, adrenal glands and gonads to the point that these glands exhaust their ability to produce enough hormones which results in hormone deficiencies. Hormone blood levels can drop to a point where pain increases and becomes even more uncontrolled and unbearable. Some hormones, especially cortisol and testosterone, are necessary for opioid receptors in the brain to function and relieve pain. Consequently, if cortisol, testosterone, or other hormones become deficient, a normally effective opioid dosage may quit working. Cortisol levels may even drop to life-threatening levels, and deaths have occurred with adrenal failure in persons with uncontrolled pain. It is interesting that Dr. Thomas Addison, who discovered adrenal failure, reported 11 cases in 1855 who died from it. Five of the 11 had uncontrolled pain and, at autopsy, showed anatomic evidence of adhesive arachnoiditis, a well-known cause of severe chronic pain.

### Cortisol Danger

When cortisol blood tests are taken from patients with uncontrolled pain, some levels will be above normal and others below. Those with high levels indicate uncontrolled pain, but the adrenal glands are keeping up with the stress. Those patients with low levels signify a potentially serious situation in that the adrenal glands are failing. This situation calls for an increase in pain control and possibly urgent cortisol replacement as illustrated by the attached brief case report.

### Case Report

*A 30-year-old man with Ehlers-Danlos Syndrome (EDS) and severe, chronic pain in multiple joints and muscle groups was referred for pain control. He was reported by family members to be lethargic, weak, non-communicative, and pale. Blood pressure was low at 100/60, and pulse was over 120 beats per minute. His cortisol level was 1.1 mg (normal range 5 to 15). This level was considered life threatening, so he was immediately started on hydrocortisone 5 mg every 4 hours. He was also started on an oral opioid, hydrocodone 10 mg every 4 hours. Within three days his lethargy, weakness, and communication had all greatly improved. Blood pressure and pulse normalized. Pain control was greatly improved, and blood cortisol was 4.0 mg/ml. Conclusion: Had hypocortisolemia not been identified, he may have expired due to adrenal failure.*

In one study, I found that among 40 patients admitted to chronic pain treatment about one-third each had high, low, or normal cortisol levels. With treatment, those in the high and low group normalized their blood levels. The major purpose for a cortisol level before treatment is to document the presence of either a high or low cortisol level, since either is hard core evidence that pain has been uncontrolled for some period of time and requires aggressive treatment.

## Prevention of Hormone Depletion

The suppression and depletion of hormones in chronic pain patients during treatment is so ubiquitous that prevention measures should be considered. Prevention of testosterone and estradiol depletion may be accomplished with DHEA supplementation (about 100 to 200 mg a day). Progesterone and allopregnanolone depletion may be prevented by pregnenolone supplementation (about 100 to 200 mg a day) since it metabolizes to these two hormones.

TABLE

Common Features of Hypocortisolemia in Pain Patients

Weakness
Weight loss
Muscle wasting
Anorexia
Hypotension
Mental apathy
Tachycardia
Pale skin
Pigmentation around skin creases or scars

## Non-Corticoid Deficiencies

A number of different hormones may be depleted by uncontrolled chronic pain. Shown here is a Table of 61 chronic pain patients who were tested with a hormone panel at the time of admission to formal chronic pain care. About 1/3rd had one or more hormone deficiencies. The finding of multiple hormonal deficiencies calls for replacement, aggressive pain control, and repeat testing.

Deficient Hormone Levels: Levels were determined by the testing laboratory.

| Deficient Hormone Levels in 61 Chronic Pain Patients Admitted to Chronic Pain Treatment* | | |
|---|---|---|
| Hormone | No. Tested | No. Low |
| ACTH | 55 | 10 (16.4%) |
| Pregnenolone | 50 | 14 (28.0%) |
| DHEA | 43 | 14 (32.6%) |
| Testosterone | 59 | 19 (32.2%) |
| Cortisol | 61 | 10 (16.4%) |
| Progesterone | 53 | 9 (17.0% |
| *Some patients had multiple deficiencies. | | |

Testing During Ongoing Treatment

The pain practitioner must constantly be on the alert for hormone deficiencies during ongoing pain treatment. Indications to do a hormone blood test and replacement are listed in the Table. Since chronic pain and its treatment with medicinals, especially opioids, may suppress various hormones, blood testing is ideally done for a panel of hormone tests that are commonly suppressed and need replacement (See Table)

TABLE

Indicators to do a Hormone Panel During Chronic Pain Treatment

- Baseline or background pain increases
- Flares more frequent and stronger
- Lack of energy and motivation
- Depression

- Mental deficiencies in memory, reading, rationalization
- Overall disease deterioration

Summary

Hormone depletion may occur with untreated chronic pain and the medicinals that treat it. (See next chapter.) Blood testing on admission to treatment as well as during treatment may be necessary to detect uncontrolled pain and a need for hormone replacement.

TABLE

Basic Hormone Test Panel
Cortisol
Pregnenolone
Estradiol
Progesterone
Testosterone
Dehydroepiandrosterone (DHEA)

## References

1. Addison T. On the constitutional and local effects of disease of the supra-renal capsules. *Samuel-Highley, London* 1855.
2. Barnes PJ. Anti-inflammatory actions of glucocorticoids: molecular mechanisms. *Clin Sci* 1998;94:557-572.
3. Blackburn-Munro G, Blackburn-Munro R. Pain in the brain: are hormones to blame? *Trends Endocrinol Metab*. 2003 Jan;14(1):20-7.
4. Chrousos GP. The hypothalamic-pituitary-adrenal axis and immune-mediated inflammation. *N Engl J Med* 1995;332:1351-1362.
5. Fischer L, Clementa JT, Tambeli CH. The protective role of testosterone in the development of temporomandibular joint pain. *J Pain* 2007;8:437-442.
6. Gibson A. The influence of endocrine hormones on the autoimmune nervous system. *J Auton Pharmaco* 1981;1:331-340.
7. Griep EN, Boersma JW, Lentjes EG, et al. Function of the hypothalamic-pituitary-adrenal axis in patients with fibromyalgia and low back pain. *J Rheumatol* 1998;25:1374-1281.
8. Harbuz MS, Perveen-Gill Z, Lightman SL, et al. A protective role for testosterone in adjuvant-induced arthritis. *Br J Rheumatol* 1995;34:1117-1122.
9. Holaday JW, Law PY, Loli HH, et al. Adrenal steroids indirectly modulate morphine and betaendorphin effects. *J Parmacol Exp Ther* 1979;208:176-183.
10. Horner HC, Packan DR, Sapolsky RM. Glucocorticoids inhibit glucose transport in

cultured hippocampal neurons and glia. *Neuroendocrinology* 1990;52:57-63.
11. Joels M, DeKloet E. Control of neuronal excitability by corticosteroid hormones. *Trends Neurosci* 1992; 15:25-30.
12. Lentjes EG, Griep EN, Boersma JW, et al. Glucocorticoid receptors, fibromyalgia, and low back pain. *Psychoneuroendocrinology* 1997;22:603-614.
13. Long JB, Holaday JW. Blood-brain barrier: endogenous modulation by adrenal-cortical function. *Science* 1985;227:1580-1583.
14. McEwen BS, Biron CA, Brunson KW, et al. The role of adrenocorticoids as modulators of immune function in health and disease: neural endocrine and immune interactions. *Brain Res Rev* 1997;23:79-133.
15. McEwen BS, de Kloet ER, Rostene W. Adrenal steroid receptors and action in the central nervous system. *Physio Rev* 1986;66:1121-1188.
16. Nakagawa H, Hosokawa R. Study of the stress response to acute pain in the awake human. *Pain Clin* 9954;7:317-324.
17. Neeck G, Federlin K, Graef V, et al. Adrenal secretion of cortisol in patients with rheumatoid arthritis. *J Rheumatol* 1990;17:24-29.
18. Orchinik M, Murray TF, Moore FL. A corticosteroid receptor in neuronal membranes. *Science* 1991;252:1848-1851.
19. Pednekar J, Mulgaonker VK. Role of testosterone on pain threshold in rats. *Indian J Physiol Pharmacol* 1995;39:423-424.

20. Shenkin HA. Effect of pain on diurnal pattern of plasma corticoid levels. *Neurology* 1964;14:1112-1117.
21. Stafford EC, Ulibarri CM, Falk JE, et al. Goadal hormone modulation of mu,kappa, and delta opioid antinociception in male and female rats. *J Pain* 2006;6:261-274.
22. Strittmatter M, Bianchi O, Ostertag D, et al. Altered function of the hypothalamic-pituitary-adrenal axis in patients with acute, chronic episodic pain. *Schmerz* 2005;19:109-116.
23. Tennant F. Intractable pain is a severe stress state associated with hypercortisolemia and reduced adrenal reserve. *Drug Alcohol Depend* 200;60:220-221.
24. Tennant F. The physiologic effects of pain on the endocrine system. *Pain Ther*. 2013 Dec;2(2):75-86.
25. Tennant F, Hermann L. Normalization of serum cortisol concentration with opioid treatment of severe chronic pain. *Pain Med* 2002;3:132-134.
26. Tennant F. Hormone abnormalities in severe, chronic pain patients who fail standard treatments. *Postgrad Med* 2015;127:1-4.

# 3. OPIOID SUPPRESSION OF HORMONES

Opioids suppress the hypothalamic and pituitary metabolism that produces multiple serum hormones. Hormonal suppression is arguably the most common and serious side effect of opioid administration. Consequently, some blood hormone levels drop, and pain may become uncontrolled and unbearable to the point that patients may bitterly complain about their well-intended opioid treatment.

A common tip off that hormones have become deficient is the chronic pain patient who takes opioids and complains that they have lost their effectiveness ("don't work like they used to"). (See attached case report.) This is especially true for patients who use long-acting opioid preparations of oxycodone and fentanyl. Methadone is also subject to loss of opioid power from hormone depletion. Especially prone to "loss of effectiveness" are patients with intrathecal opioid pumps. Multiple studies show that long-acting compared to short-acting opioid preparations are more prone to the development of hormone deficiencies.

Short-acting opioids such as hydrocodone and hydromorphone don't usually have a severe hormone suppression problem because blood levels of opioids periodically drop to zero or minimal levels so the hypothalamus and pituitary are free of suppression, can recover, and continue normal hormonal production.

When patients on opioids complain of uncontrolled pain, the blood panel tests to determine hormone deficiencies should be done (See Table in previous chapter). The most common deficiencies are testosterone and pregnenolone, but there can be deficiencies of other single or multiple hormones. All deficient hormones will require replacement and follow up blood tests. Unfortunately, opioid hormone suppression, particularly long-acting opioids, is so prevalent that regular hormone blood testing is recommended. The interval between routine testing is 3 to 6 months.

Testosterone deficiency is about as common in females as males. The replacement dose in females is about 1/4$^{th}$ of the usual male dose.

Case Report

*A 35-year-old male had severe intractable pain due to cervical neck trauma with resultant disc and nerve degeneration. He was maintained quite well on long-acting oxycodone (Oxycontin®) 60 mg twice a day and a hydrocodone-acetaminophen compound 10 mg (Norco®) for breakthrough pain. He came to his regular clinic appointment and claimed that he wasn't getting the relief from his opioids that he normally gets. On questioning he states he had been lethargic, libido had dropped, and his sleep was irregular. A presumptive diagnosis of testosterone suppression and deficiency was made, and he was given an injection of 200 mg testosterone. He provided feedback 48 hours later and stated his opioids were working again and his energy and libido were up. A blood test confirmed that his testosterone was low. Note: A testosterone injection was given here on purely clinical grounds before a blood level was done. This is perfectly acceptable as testosterone suppression with long acting and intrathecal opioids is so common and expected.*

*Testosterone Administration: Testosterone for ongoing maintenance treatment can be topical gel, patch, injection, or oral tablet. This is a practitioner's choice. Female dosage is about 1/4th of the male dosage.*

## Summary

Opioids suppress hormone levels so commonly that routine blood testing of hormone levels should be a standard component of opioid administration. Long-acting and intrathecal opioids rather than short-acting opioids are more prone to suppress hormone production. Patients on chronic opioid therapy will require hormone testing and replacement, especially when they complain of poor or inadequate pain relief after being maintained on opioid therapy.

TABLE

Quick Clinical Guide

Opioid suppression of testosterone is so common that replacement can be started on symptoms or after a low blood level. A starting injectable dosage is about 200 mg. Retest in 2 to 4 weeks.

References


1. Abs R, Verhelst J, Maeysaert J, et al. Endocrine consequences of long term intrathecal administration of opioids. *J Clin Endocrinol Metab* 2000;85:2215–22.
2. Daniell HW. DHEA deficiency during consumption of sustained-action prescribed opioids: evidence for opioid-induced inhibition of adrenal androgen production. *J Pain* 2006;7:901–7.
3. Daniel HW. Hypogonadism in men consuming sustained-action oral opioids. *J Pain* 2002;3: 377–84.
4. Daniell HW. Opioid endocrinopathy in women consuming prescribed sustained-action opioids for control of nonmalignant pain. *J Pain* 2008;9:28–36.
5. Elliott JA, Horton E, Fibuch EE. The endocrine effects of long-term oral opioid therapy: a case report and review of the literature. *J Opioid Manag* 2011;7:145–54.
6. Finch PM, Roberts LJ, Price L, et al. Hypogonadism in patients treated with intrathecal morphine. *Clin J Pain* 2000;16:251-4. 73.
7. Roberts LJ, Finch PM, Pullan PT, et al. Sex hormone suppression by intrathecal opioids: a prospective study. *Clin J Pain* 2002;18:144–8.
8. Rubinstein AL, Carpenter DM, Minkoff J. Hypogonadism in men using daily opioid therapy for non-cancer pain is associated with duration of action of opioid. Poster presentation at the 2012 Annual Meeting of the American Academy of Pain Medicine, February 23–26, 2012; Palm Springs; Abstract #229.

9. Vuong C, Van Uum SH, O'Dell LE, Lutfy K, Friedman TC. The effects of opioids and opioid analogs in animal and human endocrine systems. *Endocr Rev* 2010;31:98–132.

# 4. CORTICOSTEROIDS: ESSENTIAL IN CHRONIC PAIN CARE

Cortisol or its analogues are essential to relieve pain in many chronic painful conditions. Its best-known function is suppression of inflammation, but it has other critical biologic functions. (See Table.) For example, cortisol helps maintain the blood brain barrier, neuronal membranes, and multiple receptors in the CNS. Cortisol enhances the immune system. The corticosteroids, methylprednisolone and dexamethasone, have their own specific receptors and biologic functions in the CNS. Dexamethasone, for example, has a unique suppressive effect on viruses that invade the CNS. Methylprednisolone has been shown to have unique properties of inflammation control and regeneration of neuronal tissue in the CNS. Consequently, methylprednisolone is optimal in many pain care situations.

The natural, major corticosteroid is cortisol. About 20 to 30 mg are produced each day by the two adrenal glands. Pregnenolone and DHEA have some of the natural biologic functions of cortisol, and both of these hormones are produced in the adrenal glands, gonads, and central nervous system.

Four synthetic corticosteroids are used in pain care: hydrocortisone, prednisone, methylprednisolone, dexamethasone.

Their main clinical use is for suppression of inflammation and the pain that accompanies it. It also maintains CNS tissues. Corticosteroids reduce fatigue, improve energy, and motivation. The immune system greatly relies on cortisol to function. Corticosteroids suppress viruses such as Epstein-Barr virus (EBV).

TABLE

Biologic Uses and Functions of Corticosteroids

- Reduction of inflammation
- Viral suppression
- Maintenance of neurologic functions
- Reduction of fatigue
- Immune enhancement

The Local Injection

A long-established medical practice is the injection of a corticosteroid into a local or circumscribed anatomical area of pain. These anatomical areas have traditionally been joints and soft tissue conditions such as plantar fasciitis. The principle of bringing a corticosteroid into the painful, inflamed area has been expanded into epidural injections and spinal facets.

The local corticosteroid injection also has both diagnostic and therapeutic value. The corticosteroid is mixed in a syringe with a local anesthetic, which is about a 2-part anesthetic and 1-part corticosteroid. If the pain is caused by local inflammation, there will be immediate pain relief with the injection. In the event the injection doesn't relieve pain, it indicates that the pain is being generated elsewhere in the body and that the local pain site is likely a result of radiation.

I recall my first exposure to the merits of a local cortisone injection. I was a first-year internal medicine resident at the University of Texas Medical Branch in Galveston. I had just been assigned to the personal service of the head of the department, Dr. Raymond Gregory. He was an icon in the eyes of residents like me. On his service you worked hard and put in long hours to learn from the master. On routine hospital rounds around 9:00 PM one evening, we encountered a woman who had a respiratory condition, but she also complained profusely about lower hip pain. Much to my amazement, Dr. Gregory pulled a syringe out of his white coat pocket and told the residents, me included, to never make rounds without a syringe containing cortisol and an anesthetic. "If the injection relieves pain on the spot, the cause of pain is a local tissue issue and not a general systemic one." He gave the lady the injection and she had immediate pain relief for the first time in weeks. Today we would call her problem piriformis syndrome. The lady went to physical therapy the next day. The pain never came back. Dr. Gregory was a hero. I carried a syringe with cortisol and an anesthetic on most days for the rest of my career.

Soon after my residency in Texas, I went to active Army duty, and I encountered a general's wife with chest pain believed to be a long-standing heinous heart problem. I felt the joints that connect her ribs to her sternum. They were a little tender. Remembering Dr. Gregory's lesson, I injected her sternal joints with cortisone and her pain immediately evaporated. She had what is known as Teitzes Syndrome or costal chondritis, but to everyone else I had just cured heart disease of the wife of a general. Going forward the good general saw to it that I and my medics got whatever and whenever we needed special consideration from the upper crust.

## The Cortisone Challenge

Corticosteroids have long been a basic treatment of the inflammation and autoimmunity of rheumatoid arthritis, systemic lupus, and other autoimmune, inflammatory diseases. The major chronic pain conditions today include adhesive arachnoiditis, complex regional pain syndrome (CRPS), and advanced arthropathies and neuropathies. These conditions may or may not be associated with or caused by inflammation. Consequently, step one in treatment is to determine if a corticosteroid may be required for ongoing treatment. The best way to do this is a corticosteroid challenge to see if symptoms improve. The corticosteroid challenge can be done in a variety of ways. I like a single injection of methylprednisolone 10 to 20 mg or a 6-day methylprednisolone (Medrol®) Dose Pak.

The purpose of the challenge is to see if inflammation is suppressed and symptoms improve (i.e., less pain, more flexibility, and energy). If symptoms improve with a corticosteroid challenge, a diagnosis of current, active inflammation is determined, and an ongoing anti-inflammatory treatment regimen with a corticosteroid will be necessary.

## Ongoing Chronic Corticosteroid Treatment

Many chronic pain conditions are autoimmune and/or inflammatory based. These include adhesive arachnoiditis, fibromyalgia, systemic lupus, rheumatoid arthritis, and mixed connective tissue disease. Genetic connective tissue diseases such as Ehlers-Danlos Syndrome invariably show evidence of autoimmunity and chronic inflammation. Long-term corticosteroid therapy may be the only or best treatment in these cases. The author recommends low dose, intermittent corticosteroid therapy to avoid the well-known complications of adrenal suppression, glucose elevation, and osteoporosis. The recommended low dose, intermittent schedule, is limited to 1 to 3 times a week dosage. It is critical that days be skipped between dosages to avoid hypothalamic-adrenal suppression and other side effects. Low dosages include prednisone 5 mg, methylprednisolone 4 mg, and dexamethasone 0.5-0.75 mg. Doctors are rightfully concerned about long-term corticosteroid effects. To date, however, low dose, periodic use with skipped days between corticosteroid dosages has usually shown benefits over any risk. Early studies show that there are glucocorticoid receptors on glial cells which are the CNS cells which cause central pain (also called central sensitization). It may be that ongoing treatment with low dose; intermittent corticosteroids are the best measure to control central pain.

## Summary

A local cortisone injection is invaluable for both therapeutic and diagnostic value. A corticosteroid challenge can help determine if ongoing corticosteroid treatment is needed. Low dose, intermittent corticosteroids may be necessary for chronic pain care of some autoimmune and inflammatory conditions.

TABLE

Quick Clinical Guide

Use cortisone injection for localized pain for both diagnosis and treatment. A 6-day Medrol® Dose Pak will determine if systemic inflammation is present. Ongoing low dose intermittent corticosteroid treatment is 1 to 3 days a week.

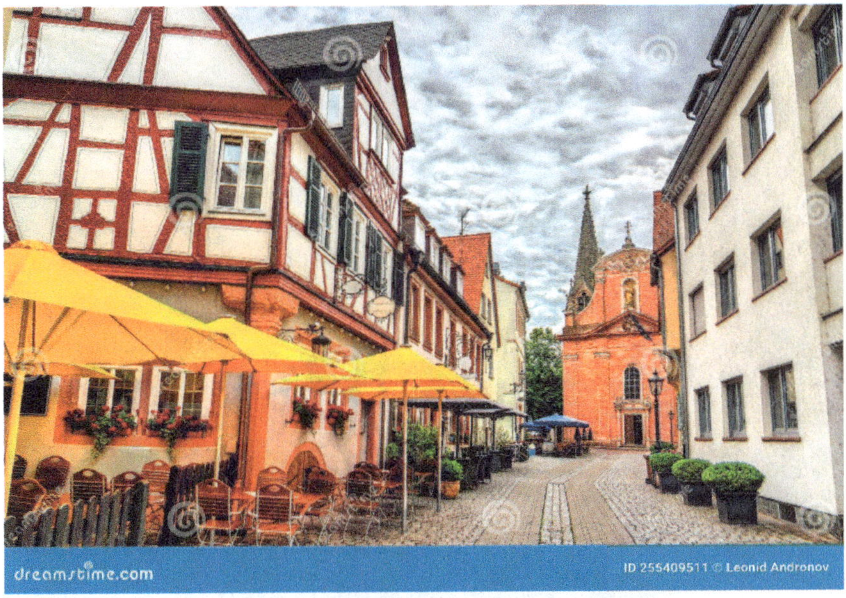


Aschaffenburg, Germany

I was assigned to the military base attached to this beautiful German town during the Cold War (late 1960's). Cortisone injections and use of low potency opioids and anabolic steroids were used extensively by US Army medical officers, such as me, on the US Army bases in Germany.

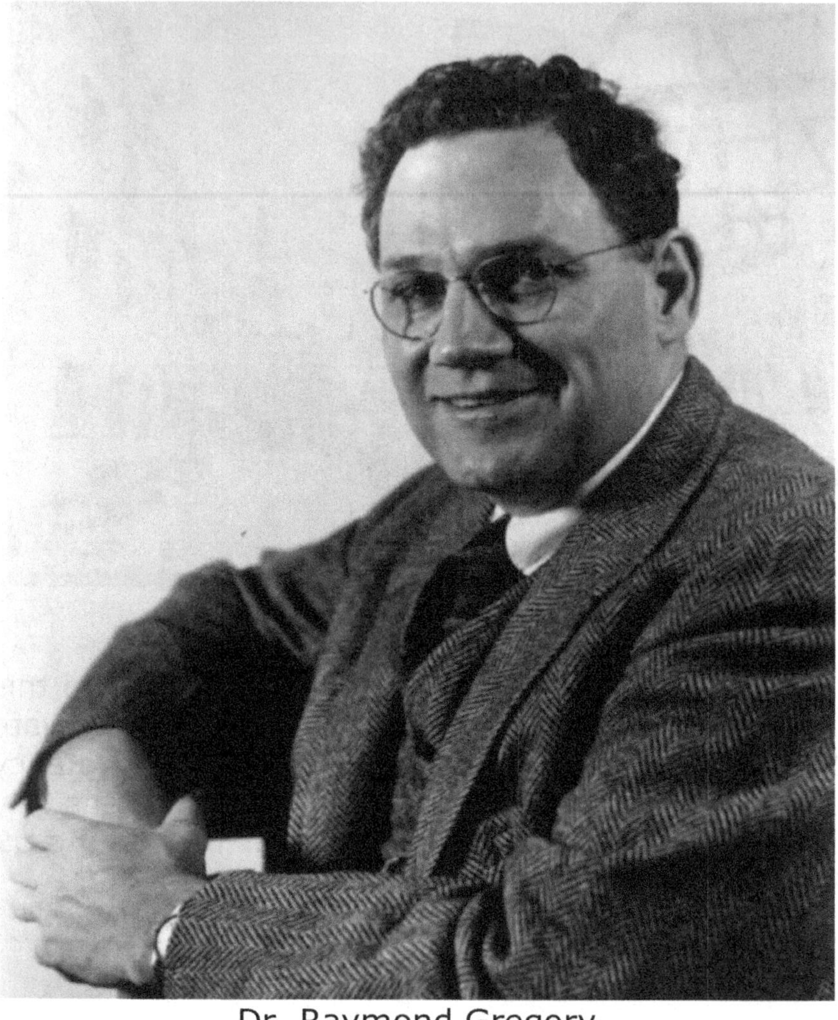

Dr. Raymond Gregory

Dr. Raymond Gregory was a prominent figure in the field of medicine, known for his contributions to both organic chemistry and pharmacology. He was born on February 20, 1901, in Beeville, Texas, and moved to Austin at the age of 15. He received his B.A. and M.A. in organic chemistry from the University of Minnesota. Dr. Gregory's career included serving as a professor and Head of the Department of Medicine at Howard University Medical School in Washington, D.C., and at the University of Arkansas School of Medicine in Litle Rock. He also held the positions of Ashbel Smith Professor of Internal Medicine and Chairman of the Department of Internal Medicine at the University of Texas Medical Branch at Galveston. Dr. Gregory passed away in 1988, leaving behind a legacy of service and education in the medical field. He taught his residents, including the author, that an injection of a corticosteroid local anesthetic was both therapeutic and diagnostic.

## References

1. Ahima R, Krozowski Z, Harlow R. Type I corticosteroid receptor-like immunoreactivity in the rat CNS: distribution and regulation by corticosteroids. *J Comp Neurol* 1991;363(3):522-538.
2. Bartholdi D, Schwab ME. Methylprednisolone inhibits early inflammatory processes but not ischemic cell death after spinal cord lesion in the rat. *Brain Res* 1995;672:177-182.
3. Bohn MC, O'Banion NK, Young DA, et al. In vitro studies of glucocorticoid effects on neurons and astrocytes. *Amer NU Acad Sci* 1994;746:243-258.
4. Bracken MB, Shepard MJ, Thorpe K, et al. A randomized, controlled trial of methylprednisolone or naltrexone in the treatment of acute spinal cord injury: results of the Second National Acute Spinal Cord Injury Study. *N Engl J Med* 1990;322:1405-1411.
5. Bracken MB, Shepard MJ, Holfor TR, et al. Administration of methylprednisolone for 24 or 48 hours of tirilazad mesylate for 48 hours in the treatment of acute spinal cord injury: results of the Third National Acute Spinal Canal Injury Randomized Controlled Trial. *JAMA* 1997;277:1597-1604.
6. Chao CC, Hu S, Close K, et al. Cytokine release from microglia: differential inhibition by pentoxifylline and dexamethasone. *J Infect Dis* 1992;166(4):842-853.
7. Chikawa T, Ikata T, Katoh S, et al. Preventive effects of lecithinized superoxide dismutase

and methylprednisolone on spinal cord injury in rats: transcriptional regulation of inflammatory and neurotrophic genes. *J Neurotrauma* 2001;18:93-103.

8. Funder JW, Sheppard K. Adrenocorticol steroids and the brain. *Am Rev Physcol* 1987;49:397-411.
9. Fu ES, Saporta S. Methylprednisolone inhibits production of interleukin-1 beta and interleukin-6 in the spinal cord following compression injury in rats. *J Neurosurg Anesth* 2005;17:82-85.
10. Fuxe K, Cintra A, Harfstrand L, et al. Central glucocorticoid receptor immunoreactive neurons: new insights into the endocrine regulation of the brain. *Am NY Acad Sci* 1987;512:362-393.
11. Fuxe K, Harfstrand A, Agnati LF, et al. Immunocytochemical studies on the localization of glucocorticoid receptors immunoreactive nerve cells in the lower brain stem and spinal cord of the male rat using a monoclonal antibody against rat liver glucocorticoid receptors. *Neurosci Lett* 1985;60(1):1-6.
12. Hall ED, Braughler JM. Effects of intravenous methylprednisolone on spinal cord lipid peroxidation and (Na',K)-ATPase activity: dose response analysis during 1st hour after contusion injury in the cat. *J Neurosurg* 1982;49:563-568.
13. Joels M, DeKloet E. Control of neuronal excitability by corticosteroid hormones. *Trends Neurosci*_1992; 15:25-30.

14. Kaur C, Wu CH, Wen CY, et al. The effects of subcutaneous injections of glucocorticoids on amoeboid microglia in postnatal rats. *Arch Histol Cytol* 1994;57(5):449-459.
15. Kiefer R, Kreutzberg GW. Effects of dexamethasone on microglial activation in vitro: selective downregulation of major histocompatibility complex class II expression in regenerating facial nucleus. *J Neuroimmunol* 1991;34(2-3):99-108.
16. Ku J, Fan G, Chen S. et al. Methylprednisolone inhibition of TNF-(alpha) expression and NF-kappaB activation after spinal cord injury in rats. *Brain Res Mol Brain Res* 1998;59:135-142.
17. Kumida M, Inaba H, Isawa E, et al. Prevention by methylprednisolone of increased circulating tumor necrosis factor-alpha levels and lung injury associated with systemic inflammatory response syndrome due to intraperitoneal hyperthermia. *Anesth Analog* 1999;88:771-776.
18. McEwen BS, de Kloet ER, Rostene W. Adrenal steroid receptors and action in the central nervous system. *Physio Rev* 1986;66:1121-1188.
19. Rabchevsky AG, Fugaccia I, Sullivan PG, et al. Efficacy of methylprednisolone therapy for the injured rat spinal cord. *J Neurosci Res* 2002;68:7-18.
20. Schverer M, Lanfumey L, Baulieu EE, et al. Neurosteroids: non-genomic pathways in neuroplasticity and involvement in neurological diseases. *Pharm & Ther*

*2018,http://doi.org/10.1016/j.pharmthera.2018.06.011*.

21. Tanaka J, Fujita H, Mostsudo S, et al. Glucocorticoid and mineralcorticoid receptors in microglial cells: the two receptor mediate differentiation effects of corticosteroids. *Glia* 1997;20:23-37.
22. Vedder L, Weiss T, Hulshoer F, et al. Glucocorticoid and mineralocorticoid receptors in rat neocorticoid and hippocampsal brain cells in culture: characterization and regulatory studies. *Brain Research* 1993;605:18-24.
23. Vielkind U, Walencewicz A, Levine JM, et al. Type II glucocorticoid receptors are expressed in oligodendrocytes and astrocytes. *J Neurosci Res* 1990;27(3):360-323.

# 5. NEUROSTEROIDS

Early in this century it was amazingly discovered that the spinal cord produces some of the same hormones that are produced in the adrenals and gonads. These include estradiol, DHEA, pregnenolone and progesterone. Cortisol and thyroid are not produced, and testosterone is probably not produced in the spinal cord, but it is a metabolite of dehydroepiandrosterone (DHEA). The four hormones that are produced are often labeled "neurosteroids" as they have a chemical structure similar to corticosteroids.

A number of astounding basic science studies have been done with spinal cord, brain injury, and pain with these four hormones. (See references.) The research models usually used were mice or rats that had a severed spinal cord and/or crush injury. Stroke models were also used. To summarize, the animal research with these neurosteroids showed that they have profound healing capability with damaged or diseased spinal cord and brain tissue. Hence, they relieve pain and may treat the underlying cause of pain.

At this time neurosteroids are the "wave of the future." To illustrate their capability, I describe here what I believe to be the most innovative and futuristic hormonal therapy program in the United States today.

Dr. Susan Sklar is an obstetrician-gynecologist in Long Beach, California. A few years ago, she was treating a middle-aged woman for perimenopausal symptoms with estrogen. This woman had one of the most rare, notorious, painful diseases one can have: "Burning Mouth Syndrome (BMS)." After a couple of months of estrogen therapy her BMS symptoms significantly improved. This was a shock because physicians who know about BMS know it rarely if ever gets better. Until Dr. Sklar, no physician anywhere had a clue as to what to do. Dr. Sklar was intrigued and decided to run neurosteroid blood tests on BMS patients. Lo and behold, she found not only estrogen deficiency but other deficiencies of neurosteroids. She developed a therapeutic program to bring all the neurosteroids into normal range. She combines her neurosteroid therapy with nutrition, anti-stress, and immunologic measures and is able to treat and bring about "near-cure" status to a previously labeled severe, disabling, untreatable disease of great suffering.

Dr. Sklar's method is simple, straight forward and probably a model for other severe painful conditions. Test for neurosteroid deficiencies and bring blood levels up to normal. In effect Dr. Sklar is putting to work what the basic science studies tell us should work.

In the subsequent chapters, I detail each neurosteroid with what I know to date. My overall impression is that every chronic pain patient should add one or more neurosteroids to their treatment plan. I'm confident that there will be more Dr. Sklar's in the future.

Dr. Susan Sklar

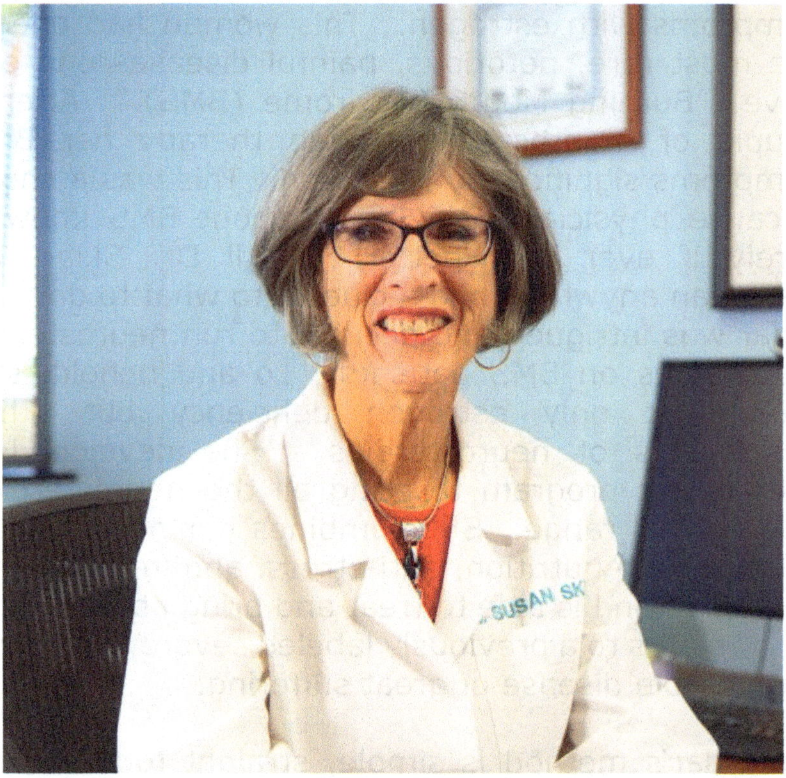


Dr. Sklar has developed an innovative futuristic treatment for Burning Mouth Syndrome that is based on neurosteroid testing and replacement.

TABLE

Neurosteroids Involved in Pain Management

- Dehydroepiandrosterone
- Estradiol
- Pregnenolone
- Progesterone

TABLE

Characteristics of Neurosteroids

- Produced inside the CNS with no pituitary or peripheral gland control
- Secreted into bloodstream and spinal fluid
- Maintain blood-brain barrier and cellular integrity
- Inhibit NMDA and GABA receptors, may enhance the latter system
- Prevent apoptosis and cellular death (neuroprotection)
- Suppress microglial cell activation and neuroinflammation
- Maintain analgesic receptors and prevent hyperalgesia
- Promote growth of damaged neurons and glial cells (neurogenesis)

## References

1. Aloisi A.M., Bonifazi M. **S**ex hormones, central nervous system and pain. *Hormones and Behavior*, 50, issue 1, 2006, 1-7
2. Compagnone NA, Mellon SH. Neurosteroids: biosynthesis and function of these novel neuromodulators. *Front Neuroendocrinol* 2000;21:1-56
3. Kilts JD, Tupler LA, Keefe FJ, et al. Neurosteroids and self-reported pain in veterans who served in the Military after September 11,2001. *Pain Med* 2010;10:1469-1476.
4. Mensah-Nyagan A.G., Meyer L., Schaeffer V., et al. Evidence for a key role of steroids in the modulation of pain**.** *Psychoneuroendocrinology*, Volume 34, Issue SUPPL. 1, 2009, S169-S177.
5. Naylor JC, Kilts JD, Szabo ST, et al. Allopregnanolone levels with self-reported pain symptoms in U.S. Iraq and Afghanistan-Era veterans: Implications for biomarkers and therapeutics. *Pain Med* 2016;17:25-32.
6. Reddy DS. Neurosteroids: endogenous role in the human brain and therapeutic potentials. *Prog Brain Res* 2010;186:13-137.
7. Schverer M, Lanfumey L, Baulieu EE, et al. Neurosteroids: non-genomic pathways in neuroplasticity and involvement in neurological diseases. *Pharm & Ther 2018,http://doi.org/10.1016/j.pharmthera.2018.06.011.*

# 6. HUMAN CHORIONIC GONADOTROPIN (HCG)

HCG is produced in large amounts by the placenta during pregnancy. It provides constant pain relief for the pregnant woman who has an expanding uterus. HCG, besides relieving pain, is the major generator of the nervous system, hair, and nails (Ectoderm) in the embryo. In non-pregnant women and men, it is regularly produced in low levels by the pituitary.

HCG has been a controversial drug as it has been used for weight control and enhanced athletic performance. Its use in weight loss has never been validated by controlled studies, and it is a banned substance in organized sports.

The author has used it extensively in intractable pain patients. Starting dosage has been 250 to 500 units 2 to 3 times a week as a sublingual preparation or injection. Patients consistently report a reduction in pain, increase in flexibility, and an overall feeling of well-being. At this time, my experience must be classified as experimental and anecdotal as there are no controlled studies.

Human chorionic gonadotropin derives its name from the fact that it was originally believed to be only produced in the placenta during pregnancy. Indeed, the common at-home pregnancy test is based on the finding of elevated HCG levels in female urine. It is now known, however, that it is also produced in the pituitary of males and females of all ages. Chemically, it is made up of two amino acid sub-units. One of the units contains amino acid sequences that are identical to FSH (follicle stimulating hormone), LH (luteinizing hormone), and TSH (thyroid stimulating hormone). Consequently, HCG, when given, stimulates the testes, ovary, thyroid, and adrenal to produce testosterone, thyroid, estradiol, progesterone and related compounds. It is this pro-hormone stimulation that gives HCG multiple clinical uses. For example, severe chronic pain patients who must take opioids and have multiple hormonal deficiencies may resolve the deficiencies by HCG's hormone-stimulating properties.

The other sub-unit of HCG also has biologic activities that assist pain patients. It increases cyclic adenosine monophosphate (cAMP) and nitric oxide (NO). cAMP is known to be a critical element in tissue production and growth while NO has important intracellular and intercellular regulatory functions. NO is known to increase blood flow. HCG receptors are found throughout the body, so it has a much greater biologic role than simply maintaining a placenta in pregnancy.

Although considerable mystery about the physiologic effects of HCG remains, it is clear that the combined effects of hormonal stimulation and enhanced tissue growth through cAMP and NO production make HCG a compelling compound for clinical use in severe, chronic pain patients.

These two case reports show that patients with severe chronic pain may benefit from HCG.

Case Report 1: A 68-year-old female had intractable pain due to severe spine degeneration. She underwent a cervical neck fusion and had lumbar spinal stenosis. Her daily opioid intake was approximately 1500 mg of morphine equivalence. Her serum testosterone was less than 20 ng/dl. She began 1000 units of HCG once a week, and later, at 30 to 60 days reported the following: increased energy, libido and sleep together with decreased pain, depression and house-bounding. Her daily opioid use dropped 30%.

Case Report 2: A 65-year-old female developed severe fibromyalgia in 1997 following a auto accident. She progressively worsened despite multiple treatments and numerous physician consults. In March 2008, she had deteriorated with constant, severe pain to the point of being bed or house bound, tachycardia over 100 per minute, insomnia, anorexia, extreme lethargy and progressive wasting, despite a daily morphine dose equivalence of approximately 3500 mg. Serum testosterone concentration was less than 12 ng/dl. As a last option, she was started on HCG, 500 to 1000 units three times a week. Within a week she began to have more energy, appetite, lowered pulse rate, and less pain. After a year's treatment she stated her pain was approximately 50% improved and her daily opioid intake has dropped to about 140 mg morphine equivalence per day.

HCG can be injected or formulated (compounded) as a sublingual or buccal preparation. Patients are given one or two trial dosages of 250 to 500 USP units. If patients believe they experience positive effects with libido, energy or pain relief, they can be given a 30 to 60-day course of 1 to 3 weekly dosages. My experience is that most patients report extraordinary results. A few patients report no effects with HCG. Acne or hair falling out has occurred in some females and necessitated stopping HCG or reducing the dosage. No other significant side effects have been observed. Dosages can be raised as needed. Some patients report immediate pain relief that lasts several hours. Other patients report longer term effects such as a reduction in baseline pain, longer intervals between flares, and/or less severe flares.

HCG has been used by athletes to enhance performance since at least the early 1970's. Some states now classify HCG as an anabolic steroid and/or classify it as a controlled substance in an attempt to limit its non-medical use. Ethical pain practitioners must guard against any attempts by teenagers or other athletes to obtain it for non-medical purposes.

A book entitled, "The Practical Use of Anabolic Steroids with Athletes," was written by Robert Kerr, MD in 1982 before anabolic steroids became a controversial banned substance in sports. Dr. Kerr had been treating athletes with anabolic steroids for over 15 years prior to writing his book. The book was widely distributed and followed in the sports world. The book is now highly sought after as an "underground bible" on anabolic steroids. Dr. Kerr stated that HCG built muscles and other tissues by virtue of simultaneously raising testosterone levels and cAMP and NO. Furthermore, he found that HCG built blood vessels. Body builders wish to show off large blood vessels in their arms in competition and can achieve the desired appearance with HCG. Since HCG will enhance athletic performance there is great bias in using the hormone even for legitimate medical purposes. This is an ignorant bias. The only way a drug can enhance athletic performance is to make body tissues, including nerves, muscles, ligaments, and other tissues stronger and more pain resistant. Some severe chronic pain conditions such as adhesive arachnoiditis, pudendal neuropathy, cervical neuropathy, and EDS need to be given trials of HCG because of the need to enhance tissue regeneration. Clearly HCG is an underused hormonal therapy in severe chronic pain patients.

TABLE

Quick Clinical Guide

Start sublingual or injectable HCG at 250 to 500 units on 2 or 3 days a week. Can increase dosage as needed.

## References


1. Braunstein GD. Human Chorionic Gonadotropin in *William's Textbook of Endocrinology*. 10th Ed. Saunders, Philadelphia. 2003; pp 800-803.
2. Kerr P, Human Chorionic Gonadotropin in *The Practical Use of Anabolic Steroids with Athletes*. 1982. San Gabriel, CA pp 75-79.
3. Lei ZM, Rao CV. Neural actions of luteinizing hormone and human chorionic gonadotropin. *Seminar Reprod Med* 2001;19:103-109.
4. Lei ZM, Rao CV, Kornyei JL, et al. Novel expression of human chorionic gonadotropin/luteinizing hormone receptor gene in brain. *Endocrin* 1993;132:2262-2270.
5. Lei ZM, Rao CV. Novel presence of luteinizing hormone/human chorionic gonadotropin (HCG) receptors and the down-regulating action of HCG on gonadotropin releasing hormone gene expression in immortalized hypothalamic GTI-7 neurons. *Mol EndocrinoI* 1994;8:1111-1121.
6. Li X, Lei ZM, Rao CV. Human chorionic gonadotropin down-regulates the expression of gonadotropin releasing hormone receptor gene in GTI-7 neurons. *Endocrin* 1996;137:899-904.
7. Lukacs H, Hiatt ES, Lei ZM, et aI. Peripheral and intracerebroventricular administration of human chorionic gonadotropin alters several hippocampus associated behaviors in cycling female rats. *Hor and Behav* 1995;29:42-58.
8. Matura S, Okashi M, Chen HC, et al. Physiochemical and Immunological Characterization of an HCG-Like Substance from Human Pituitary Glands. *Nature* 1980; 286: 740-741.

9. Odell WD, Griffin J. Pulsatile secretion of Human Chorionic Gonadotropin in Normal Adults. *N Engl J Med* 1987; 317: 1688-1692.
10. Patil AA, Nagaraj MP. The effect of human chorionic gonadotropin (HCG) on functional recovery of spinal cord sectioned rats. *ACTA Neurochir* 1983 ;69:205-218.
11. Tennant F. Human chorionic gonadotropin in pain treatment. *Prac Pain Manag* 2009;9:44-46.

# 7. WELCOME BACK THE OLD-FASHIONED ESTROGEN SHOT

In addition to corticosteroids, estrogen has been the other hormone that has a long history in pain care. Its use is historically one of empirical use. For example, literally millions of women took an estrogen shot in the last century for post-menopausal symptoms including pain. A misinformed, erroneous report on estrogen in 2002, however, essentially sent the use of estrogen for pain and menopause care to the grave. Recently, the folly and falsehood of this report have been discovered and retracted. Estrogen use for menopause and pain care are on the way back.

The author's first encounter with the "old-fashioned" estrogen shot is given here to illustrate an old practice that is coming back in vogue.

*"Hello, my name is Nellie. I like to meet all the medical students who come to our town to study with our fine doctors. The year was 1966 and I was a senior medical student at the University of Kansas Medical School. In those years, a senior medical student spent a month with rural doctors in a rural town. My town was Norton, a farm community in*

*northwest Kansas, of a few thousand population. Nellie was almost a duplicate of my grandmother, who was also a lifetime farmer. She wore a colorful, flowered dress fashioned from feed sacks, wore a leather shawl, and laced up oxfords. Her demeanor was positive and proud to have been a farming success on the prairie. Her hands were deeply tanned with knuckles swollen and bent. They called these "farmer hands" rather than osteoarthritis. Over the years, farmers carry buckets, shuck corn, milk cows, drive tractors, trucks, and horses thanks to strong hands. Nellie proceeded to tell me what a great community Norton was and how fortunate I was to be training with their doctors. I asked her why she had come to the clinic. She said, "Doc gives me an estrogen shot every month. Without estrogen the pain in these old hands wouldn't let me sleep much or tend to the farm." In summary, we should heed Nellie's message. An estrogen shot may do wonders. What happened to the "old-fashioned" estrogen shot? It essentially disappeared in recent years. It is a sad and pathetic story, but the "old-fashioned" shot is coming back.*

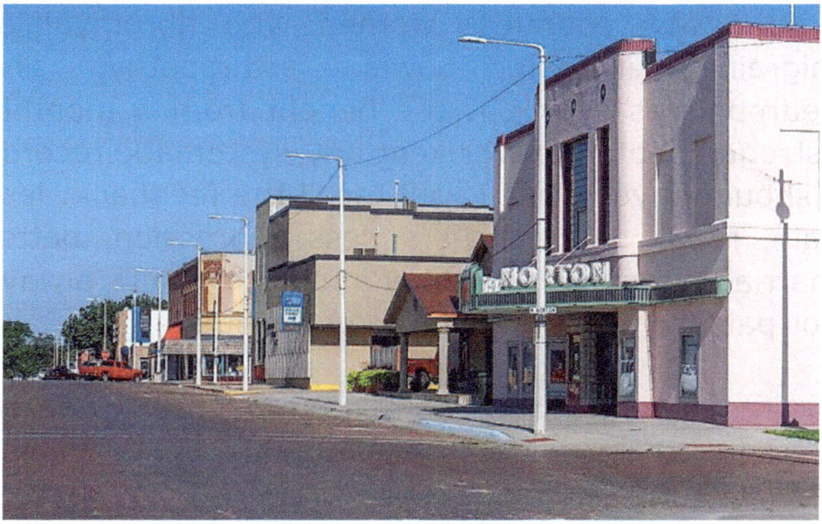


Norton, Kansas, a rural town in northwest Kansas that introduced estrogen for "Farmer's Hands" to the author.

Starting with "Farmer's Hands" in Norton, Kansas, I became a fan and practitioner of the estrogen shot or its equivalent for painful conditions. I began my pain clinic in West Covina, California in 1976. The initial mission was to provide care primarily for post-polio neuropathies and metastatic cancer. Over time, however, I began receiving referrals for all types of pain conditions from local practitioners who couldn't manage their pain patients. I operated my clinic for 40 years until I retired from clinical practice to do full-time research and education on chronic pain conditions. During this time, I observed and/or treated several hundred female patients with the old-fashioned estrogen shot or alternately 1 or 2 days a week with an oral estrogen. The clinic offered the estrogen shot to any female who wanted one. Over time I saw countless women with fibromyalgia, migraine, irritable bowel, arthropathy, and neuropathies seek out the benefit from a monthly estrogen shot. I never kept any systematic records ("should have"), but I well recall the feedback: less pain, fewer pain relievers, less depression, better marriage, feel better. What's more, my bills always got paid from women who took estrogen.

Interestingly, word spread that our pain clinic offered estrogen to any woman who wanted to take it. I also operated methadone clinics for over 25 years, and many female heroin addicts asked for estrogen. Reason: they claimed their craving for opioids diminished with the old-fashioned monthly estrogen shot in addition to relieving their pain conditions.

Unfortunately, a terrible event took place in 2002. In one of the great fraudulent, deceitful, and harmful medical events of modern medicine, we lost the "old-fashioned estrogen shot" as well as humane, effective treatment of menopause. Practitioners and chronic pain patients should know what happened to the "old-fashioned estrogen shot", and why it is now coming back.

### *What Happened in 2002?*

*In July 2002, preliminary data from the Women's Health Initiative (WHI) were published in JAMA (Journal of American Medical Association), stating that combined hormone therapy (estrogen and progestin) increased the risk of breast cancer, stroke, and pulmonary embolism. Major media outlets interpreted early signals from the study as definitive danger, and the announcement led to an instant and dramatic decline in the use of hormone therapy. Media lambasted estrogen without mercy (See compendium of headlines.*

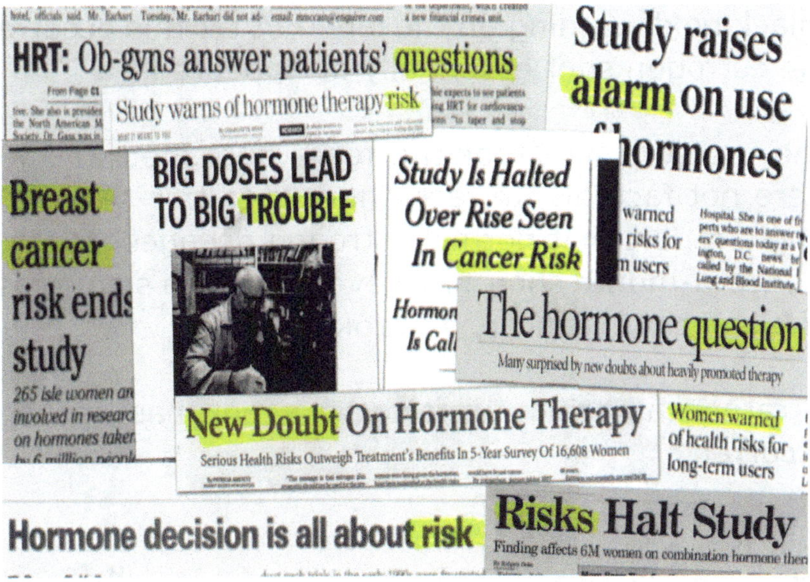
HRT: Ob-gyns answer patients' questions
Study warns of hormone therapy risk
Study raises alarm on use
Breast cancer
BIG DOSES LEAD TO BIG TROUBLE
Study Is Halted Over Rise Seen In Cancer Risk
The hormone question
Many surprised by new doubts about heavily promoted therapy
New Doubt On Hormone Therapy
Serious Health Risks Outweigh Treatment's Benefits In 5-Year Survey Of 16,608 Women
Women warned of health risks for long-term users
Hormone decision is all about risk
Risks Halt Study
Finding affects 6M women on combination hormone

Compendium of headlines after the frightening and misinformed estrogen report of 2002. Estrogen treatments went into hibernation after this misguided but well-intended report.

*Women who had been sleeping well for the first time in years suddenly poured their medications into the trash. Pharmacies fielded calls from panicked patients demanding immediate discontinuation. Primary care doctors, most of whom had never been trained deeply in menopause management, told their patients to "stop now and ask questions later."*

*Women did stop, and many suffered in silence for the next 20 years.*

The US Food and Drug Administration (FDA) put a "black box" warning on the label. After this occurred the estrogen shot essentially disappeared.

The problem was that the fears published in 2002 were not factual. In fact, there is to this day not a single report that normal estrogen dosages, such as a once-a-month shot, have ever caused a single case of blood clots, cancer, or stroke.

A rather amazing turnaround event has recently occurred.

*On Nov. 10, 2025, the FDA announced that it is removing the broad "black box" warnings referencing risks of cardiovascular disease, breast cancer, and probable dementia from hormone replacement therapy products for menopause.*

*When FDA Commissioner Dr. Marty Makary spoke publicly about the shift, he didn't mince words. He said the media had frightened women away from a potentially life-changing therapy, and he noted the difference between estrogen-only therapy and synthetic combination regimens. He acknowledged, openly, that the fear machine" had begun long before the scientific data had been fully understood.*

*He also said something that struck many women deeply: "After 23 years of dogma, the FDA is stopping the fear that has steered women away from this life-saving treatment."*

*For many women with chronic pain, that sentence felt like a validation they had waited half a lifetime to hear.*

Pain practitioners and chronic pain patients are great beneficiaries of this admission of gross errors. The estrogen shot can come back and the painful aberrations of menopause and chronic pain conditions can again be treated.

Should the estrogen shot or other formulation of estrogen be used today? In my opinion, yes. There are basic science studies in which estrogen clearly has great pain relief and regenerative properties. (See references.) For example, estrogen activates spinal opioid receptors. Also, estrogen is produced in the spinal dorsal horn neurons. Studies also validate the use of estrogen in relief of joint pain. Since it is now permissible and available without legal entrapment, an "old-fashioned" estrogen shot should be given a trial by every woman with severe chronic pain who wants it. What is there to lose? There is much to gain.

At this time there are no reports of estrogen given systematically to chronic pain patients. Estrogen is just now starting to again be used by innovative pain practitioners. (See Dr. Sklar in a previous chapter.) One reason estrogen, per se, has not been used in pain care is that both DHEA and HCG raise estrogen blood levels. It is also possible that colostrum and deer antler velvet raise estrogen levels. The use of DHEA and HCG is simply and safely done, and their major therapeutic effects are likely to be related to increased estrogen blood levels. Pain practitioners have a choice. They can give the monthly shot, low dose oral administration, or provide DHEA or HCG which raises estrogen levels.

TABLE

Quick Clinical Guide Estrogen Administration

- Monthly injection, 10 to 20 mg
- Oral estrogen 3 days a week, 1 to 5 mg
- DHEA, 200 mg in AM and PM
- HCG 250 to 500 units, 3 times a week

References

1. Cutolo M, Capellino S, Suli A, et al. Estrogens and autoimmune disease. *Ann NY Acad Sci* 2006;1089:982-988.
2. Cutolo M. Estrogen metabolites: increasing evidence for their role in rheumatoid arthritis and systemic lupus erythematosus. *J Rheumatol* 2004;31:419-421.
3. Dawson-Basoa M, Gintzler AR. Estrogen and progesterone activate spinal kappa-opiate receptor analgesic mechanisms. *Pain* 1996;64:508-615.
4. Evrard HC, Balthazart J. Rapid regulation of pain by estrogen synthesized in spinal dorsal horn neurons. *J Neurosci* 2004;24:7225-7229.
5. Green PS, Bishop J, Simpkins JW. 17 alpha-estradiol exerts neuroprotective effects on SK-N-SH cells. *J Neurosci* 1997;17:511-515.
6. Hunter DA, Barr GA, Amador N, et al. Estradiol-induced antinociceptive responses on formalin-induced nociception are independent of COX and HPA activation. *Synapse* 2011;65:643-651.

# 8. PREGNENOLONE

Every pain practitioner should know some of the fascinating history of pregnenolone. It is also one of the most underutilized medicinals in chronic pain care.

Pregnenolone is derived from cholesterol, and it is the precursor of all the hormones produced in the adrenals or spinal cord. (See hormonal pathway in Chapter One) During World War II, it was tested in factories and found to reduce fatigue and enhance energy and work productivity. The idea was to increase productivity during World War II. The author has observed many persons who take pregnenolone, and these performance enhancement traits are commonly experienced. Take a dose and you may feel energized. Also, in the 1940's, pregnenolone, along with implanted cortisone tablets, were the major treatment for rheumatoid arthritis. The dosage of pregnenolone required for pain relief was 400 to 600 mg a day. Pregnenolone use became almost extinct when prednisone was developed and marketed in the early 1950's. Prednisone seemed quicker acting and was easier to prescribe, but some observers at the time felt it was no more effective than pregnenolone. Big pharma marketing was alive and well in the early 1950's, so prednisone was successfully sold as a pregnenolone and hydrocortisone substitute.

In persons who cannot take a corticosteroid, the author recommends pregnenolone 200 mg in AM and PM. (Just like in 1945) To help determine if pregnenolone may assist chronic pain patients the author conducted two studies. In the first study 18 intractable pain patients with poor pain control were identified who had low serum pregnenolone levels at the start of their pain treatment. Ninety days after entering treatment and after achieving some stabilization of pain, a repeat serum pregnenolone was determined. Serum pregnenolone rose to normal in 14 of the 18 (77.8%) and mean serum levels rose from 13.6 to 50.1 ng/ml (p<.oo1). This study indicates that pain control reduces stress on the pituitary-adrenal axis so normal levels of pregnenolone could be produced. The study also highlights that a low serum pregnenolone level likely means that pain is poorly controlled.

A second study involved 36 intractable pain patients who were enrolled in an ongoing treatment program. All used opioids plus a variety of neuropathic and anti-inflammatory drugs. Chewable 10 mg pregnenolone tablets were offered to the 36 patients. They were allowed to chew as many as they needed or wanted to achieve better pain control and reduction of other symptoms. At the end of 90 days, each participant was questioned as to whether pregnenolone helped their pain control and other symptoms including but not limited to energy, sleep, mental concentration, and less suffering or depression. Twenty-six of 36 (72.2%) reported improved pain relief and other symptoms. A total of 29 of 36 (80.6%) desired to continue pregnenolone after 90 days. No significant drop in opioid or other medications occurred. The dosage ranged widely from 10 to 120 mg a day. This study suggests that pregnenolone may improve pain control and other symptoms but did not show a tendency to reduce opioid use.

One of the major attributes of pregnenolone is that it metabolizes to all other adrenal and gonadal hormones including progesterone and allopregnanolone. Both hormones appear to have potent pain relief properties. Arguably, pregnenolone could or should be a supplement for every chronic pain patient since it tends to minimize deficiencies of multiple hormones.

Interestingly, pregnenolone has never found a role in athletic enhancement but it clearly enhances mental and intellectual functions. This means it affects the glial cells, neurons, and receptors in the central nervous system. Pregnenolone is worthy of trials in chronic pain patients who have central pain or central sensitivity.

TABLE

Quick Clinical Guide Pregnenolone Administration

- General supplement to prevent hormone deficiencies, 100 to 200 mg a day
- Alternative to corticosteroids, 200 mg in AM and PM

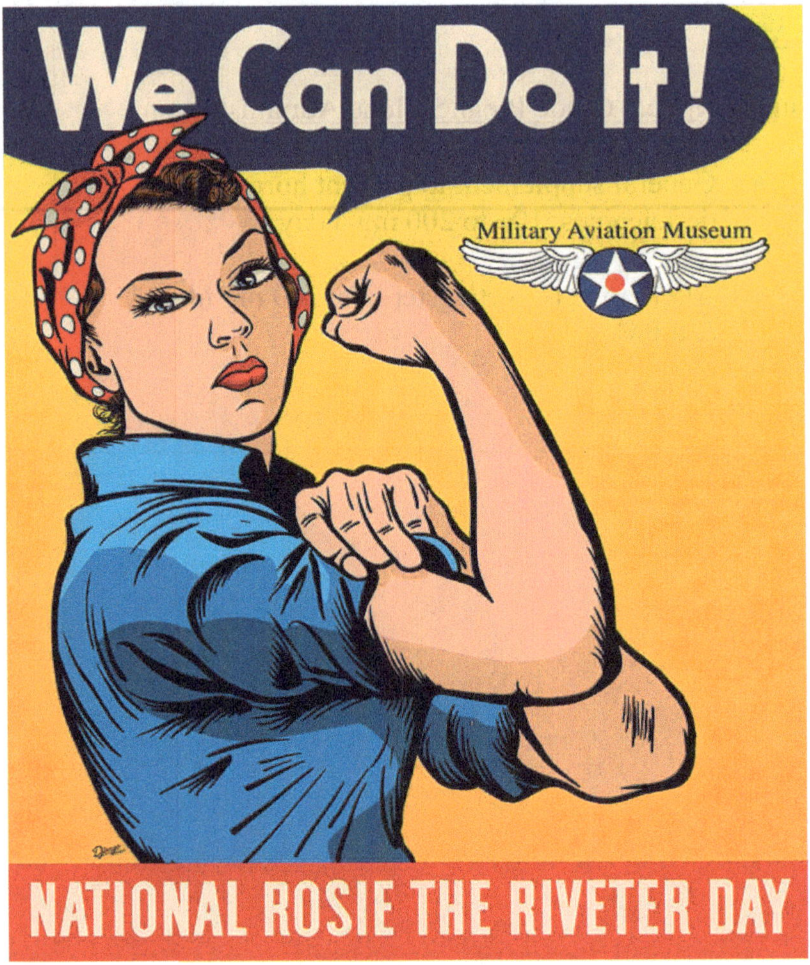


During World War II, pregnenolone was taken in factories to increase productivity. It was found to reduce fatigue and enhance energy.

References

1. Ceccon M, Runbaugh G, Vincini S. Distinct effect of pregnenolone sulfate on NMDA receptor subtypes. *Neuropharm* 2001;40:491-500.
2. Flood JF, Morley JE, Roberts E. Memory-enhancing effects in male mice of pregnenolone and steroids metabolically derived from it. Proc Natl Acad Sci 1992;89:1567-1571.
3. Freeman H, Pincus G, Bachrach S, et al. Therapeutic efficacy of delta 5 pregnenolone in rheumatoid arthritis. *JAMA* 1950;143:338-344.
4. Guth L, Zhang Z, Roberts E. Key role for pregnenolone in combination therapy that promotes recovery after spinal cord injury. *Proc Natl Acad Sci* 1994;91:12308-12312.
5. Henderson E, Weinberg M, Wright WA. Pregnenolone. *J Clin Endo* 1950;10:455-474.
6. McGavack TH, Chevalley J, Weissberg 1. The use Delta 5 pregnenolone in various clinical disorders. *J Clin EndocrinoI* 1951;11(6):559-577.
7. Morlin R, Young J, Corpechot C, et al. Neurosteroids: pregnenolone in human sciatic nerves. *Proc Natl Acad Sci* 1992;98:6790-793.
8. Pincus G, Hoagland H. Effects of administered pregnenolone on fatiguing psychomotor performance. *Aviation Med* 1944;April:98-115.
9. Pincus G, Hoagland H. Effects on industrial production of the administration of delta 5 pregnenolone to factory workers. *I Psychosomatic Med* 1945;7:342-346.
10. Shen W, Mennerick S, Covey DF, et al. Pregnenolone sulfate modulates inhibitory synaptic transmission by enhancing $GABA_a$

receptor desensitization. *J Neuroscience* 2000;20:3571-3579.
11. Vallee M, Mayo W, Le Moal M. Role of pregnenolone, dehydroepiandrosterone and their sulfate esters on learning and memory in cognitive aging. *Brain Res Brain Res Rev* 2001 ;37(1-3):301-12.

# 9. DEHYDROEPIANDROSTERONE (DHEA)

DHEA and its sulfate ester (DHEA-1) are among the most ubiquitous hormones in the human body. DHEA is made in the adrenals, gonads, and spinal cord. It is the most studied of the neurosteroids. It has multiple attributes in chronic pain patients, and it should arguably be given a trial in all cases of severe chronic pain for these two reasons:

1. It metabolizes to estradiol and testosterone and possibly nandrolone.

2. It has neuroregenerative properties

DHEA is the one neuroregenerative hormone that has been subjected to double-blind, controlled studies. These have been done on patients with systemic lupus erythematosus (SLE) who were severe enough to require corticosteroids and autoimmune agents. A daily dosage of 200 mg was found to reduce pain flares and the chronic symptoms of baseline pain, lethargy, and depression.

DHEA may be found deficient in blood specimens taken from patients whose pain is poorly controlled. It should be replaced in this situation.

The attributes of DHEA include neuroregeneration and neuroprotection of both neurons and the glial cells that are responsible for constant central (often called neuropathic) pain. DHEA also has anti-inflammatory properties and enhances the innate immune system. It has been shown to reduce interleukins, especially IL-10.

Although laboratories may differ, an adequate normal range is usually about 45 to 270 ug/dl, some investigators recommend levels be kept above 200 ug/dl.

Given the documented benefits of DHEA, the author recommends a daily dose of DHEA be given a trial in almost all chronic pain patients. It can be used as a supplement to raise estradiol and testosterone, and/or used to enhance neuroregeneration and reduce pain. The starting dosage is 200 mg a day. This dosage can be increased to 400 mg a day given in divided dosages. The only side effects reported have been acne or loss of hair which calls for a reduced daily dosage.

TABLE

Quick Clinical Guide DHEA Administration

- Prevention of estradiol and testosterone deficiencies, 100 to 200 mg a day
- Promote neuroregeneration, 200 mg in AM and PM

TABLE

DHEA Attributes in Pain Treatment

- Reduce inflammation
- Enhances innate immune system
- Viral control
- Stimulates gamma aminobutyric acid and N-methyl-d-aspartate receptors for pain relief
- Decrease insulin resistance
- Neuroprotective and neuroregenerative effect on glial cells
- Increase testosterone and estradiol levels

References

1. Bastianetto S, Ramassamy C, Poirier J, et al. Dehydroepiandrosterone (DHEA) protects hippocampal cells from oxidative stress-induced damage. *Brain Res Mol Brain Res* 1999;66:35-41.
2. Baulieu EE, Robel P. Dehydroepiandrosterone (DHEA) and dehydroepiandrosterone sulfate (DHEAS) as neuroactive neurosteroids. *Proc Natl Acad Sci* 1998;95:4089-4091.
3. Boudou P, Sobngwi E, Ibrahim F, et al. Hyperglycemia acutely decreases circulating dehydroepiandrosterone levels in healthy men. *Clin Endocrinol* (Oxf) 2006 Jan;64(1):46-52.
4. Chang DM, Chu SJ, Chen HC, et al. Dehydroepiandrosterone suppresses interleukin 10 synthesis in women with systemic lupus erythematosus. *Ann Rheum Dis* 2004;63:1623-1620.
5. Daniell HW. DHEAS deficiency during consumption of sustained-action prescribed opioids: evidence for opioid-induced inhibition of adrenal androgen production. *J Pain*. 2006 Dec;7(12):901-7.
6. Dhatariya K, Bigelow ML, Nair KS. Effect of dehydroepiandrosterone replacement on insulin sensitivity and lipids in hypoadrenal women. *Diabetes* 2005;Mar;54(3):765-769.
7. Diamond P, Cusan L, Gomez JL, et al. Metabolic effects of 12-month percutaneous dehydroepiandrosterone replacement therapy in postmenopausal women. *J Endocrinol* 1996 Sept;150 Suppl:S43-50.
8. DiSanto E, Fodde MC, Ricciardi-Castognol P, etal. DHEAS inhibits TNF production in monocytes,

astrocytes and microglial cells. *Neuroimmunomod* 1996;3:285-288.

9. Immamura M, Prausad C. Modulation of GABA-gated chloride ion influx in the brain by dehydroepiandrosterone and its metabolites. *Biochem Biophys Res Commun* 1998;24:243-(3):771-115.
10. Jellinek PH, Kaufmann M, Gottfied-Blackmore A, et al. Selective conversion by microglial of dehydroepiandrosterone to 5-androstenedial-asteroid with inherent estrogenic properties. *J Steroid Biochem Mol Biol* 2007;107:156-162.
11. Karishma KK, Herbert J. Dehydroepiandrosterone (DHEA) stimulates neurogenesis in the hippocampus of the rat, promotes survival of newly formed neurons and prevents corticosterone induced suppression *Eur J Neurosci* 2002;16:445-453.
12. Lazardis J, Charalampopoulos I, Alexaki V, et al. Neurosteroid dehydroepiandrosterone interacts with nerve growth factor (NGF) receptors preventing neuronal apoptosis. *Plos Biol* 2001;9(4):e1001051.
13. Shealy CN, Cody RK, Cox RH, et al. DHEA deficiency in patients with chronic pain and depression. *J Neuro Orthopedic Med & Surg* 1996;17(1):7-9.
14. Shealy CN. A review of dehydroepiandrosterone (DHEA). *Integ Physiol Behav Sci* 1995;30(4):308-313.
15. Shelay CN, Myss CM, Cody RK, et al. Electrical stimulation raises DHEA and improves diabetic neuropathy. *Stress Med* 1995;11:215-217.
16. Surrey C, Vela J, Garcia-Tornadir I, et al. Dehydroepiandrosterone (DHEA) modulates

GHRH, somatostatin, and angiotensin 11 action at the pituitary level. *J Endocrin* 2005;185:165-172.

17. Villareal DT, Holoszy JO. Effect of DHEA on abdominal fat and insulin action in elderly women and men: a randomized controlled trial. *JAMA* 2004;Nov 10;292(18):2243-2248.
18. Vallee M, Mayo W, Le Moal M. Role of pregnenolone, dehydroepiandrosterone and their sulfate esters on learning and memory in cognitive aging. *Brain Res Brain Res Rev* 2001;37(1-3):301-312.
19. Yamashita R, Saito T, Satoh S, et al. Effects of dehydroepiandrosterone on gluconeogenic enzymes and glucose uptake in human hepatoma cell line, HepG2. *Endocr J* 2005 Dec;52(6):727-733.

# 10. PROGESTERONE

Multiple basic science studies have established that progesterone has profound healing and neuroregeneration capabilities after a stroke or trauma to the brain or spinal cord. Its metabolite, allopregnanolone, was found to be low in studies of military men who had chronic pain and who returned from Middle East conflicts. These studies suggested that adequate pain relief has dependency on adequate serum levels of progesterone and allopregnanolone. Unfortunately, no studies were done to determine which came first. Did low levels of allopregnanolone precede or follow the development of pain. Despite these studies in military persons with chronic pain, neither progesterone nor allopregnanolone has established a niche in chronic pain care.

Progesterone and its metabolite, allopregnanolone, are both produced in the central nervous system. Multiple studies show that these hormones are associated with neuroprotection, neuroregeneration, and myelin formation. (See attached references) Animal studies of spinal cord crush injuries show that progesterone accelerates the healing process.

Enhanced recovery after stroke with progesterone is documented.

The author uses progesterone in two circumstances:

1. Low serum levels indicating a deficiency.

2. Patients who develop pain and other symptoms after a spinal tap, epidural injection, blood patch, or spine surgery. A dose of 100 to 200 mg a day for 7 to 10 days is used.

No systematic data has yet been collected, but preliminary observations by the author are that progesterone given with methylprednisolone may be effective in preventing adhesive arachnoiditis if symptoms develop after a medical procedure.

The only clinical study that we can identify is a small open trial done by the author. Nine severe chronic pain patients were started on 10 mg of medroxyprogesterone. The dosage was raised to 20 to 40 mg a day over a period of 90 days. Six of the nine patients reduced their pain and reported an increase in energy, libido, and mental ability. Pain reduction was in the range of 20 to 30 percent, but daily opioid dosage was not appreciably reduced.

One of the reasons that progesterone has not yet been used in pain care is that pregnenolone metabolizes to progesterone and allopregnanolone. Pregnenolone is an over-the-counter hormone that will raise progesterone and allopregnanolone blood levels. The pregnenolone supplement dosage is 100 to 200 mg a day.

Progesterone production may be reduced by both severe chronic pain and opioid administration. It should be replaced when found, by blood tests, to be deficient. Progesterone administration for ongoing chronic pain urgently needs trials.

TABLE

Quick Clinical Guide Progesterone Administration

- Replacement with low serum level, 100 mg a day
- Treatment of post-spinal tap, epidural injection, or surgery pain and neurologic symptoms, 100 to 200 mg for 10 days

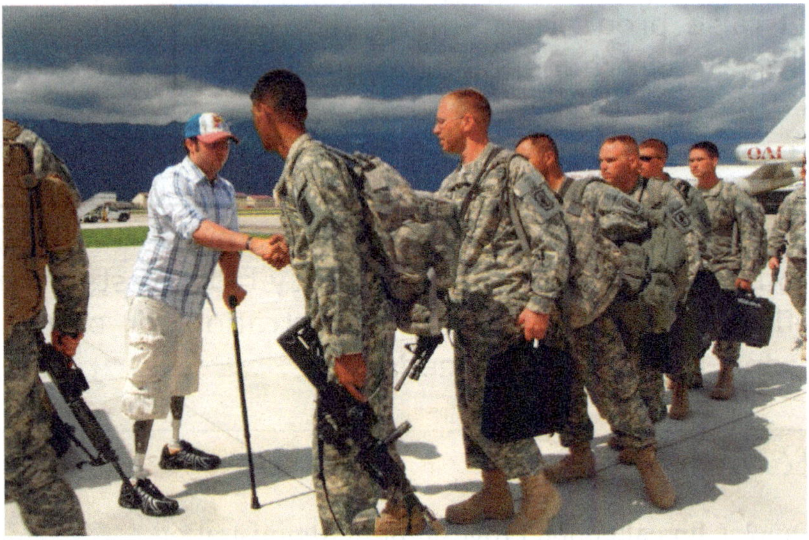

Soldiers returning from Middle East conflicts who had chronic pain were found to have low serum levels of allopregnanolone, a metabolite of pregnenolone and progesterone. It was undetermined if the low levels were the cause or result of the pain.

References

1. Coronel MF, Labomlorda F, Roig P, et al. Progesterone prevents allodynia after experimental spinal cord injury. J of Pain 2011;12:71-83.
2. Djeball M, Guo Q, Pertus EH, et al. The neurosteroids progesterone and allopregnanolone reduce cell death, gliosis, and functional deficits after traumatic brain injury in rate. *J Neurotrauma* 2005;22:106-118.
3. He J, Evans CO, Hoffman SW, et al. Progesterone and allopregnanolone reduce inflammatory cytokines after traumatic brain injury. *Exp Neuro* 2004;189:404-412.
4. Kilts JD, Tupler LA, Keefe FJ, et al. Neurosteroids and self-reported pain in veterans who served in the Military after September 11,2001. *Pain Med* 2010;10:1469-1476.
5. Naylor JC, Kilts JD, Szabo ST, et al. Allopregnanolone levels with self-reported pain symptoms in U.S. Iraq and Afghanistan-Era veterans: Implications for biomarkers and therapeutics. *Pain Med* 2016;17:25-32.
6. Roglio I, Bianchi R, Gotti S, et al. Neuroprotective effects of dehydroprogesterone and progesterone in an experimental model of nerve crush injury. *Neurosci* 2008 Aug 26;155(3):673-685.
7. Tennant F. Clinical trial of progesterone for intractable, central pain. *Presented at Amer Acad Pain Med*, Palm Springs, CA 2012.
8. Webster KM, Wright DK, Sun M, et al. Progesterone treatment reduces neuroinflammation, oxidative stress and brain

damage and improves long-term outcomes in a rat model of repeated mild traumatic brain injury. *J Neuroinflammation* 2015 Dec 18;12-238.

# 11. ANABOLIC STEROIDS

Anabolic steroids (AS) are included in this book because more and more chronic pain patients are being identified in a stage of wasting or catabolic deterioration, and in need of palliative care. Also, more patients have multiple painful conditions. A major labeled clinical indication for anabolic steroids is for wasting states. In pain care, we are especially witnessing severe wasting and deterioration in persons who have a genetic connective tissue disease such as Ehlers-Danlos syndrome and those with autoimmune disorders that may or may not be related to a viral reactivation syndrome. For whatever reason, there seems to be an increasing number of chronic pain patients who are deteriorating into a dysfunctional, bed or house bound state. Families complain about the patient's significant deterioration and progressive inability to carry out activities of daily living. For lack of a better description, families often say their loved one seems to be "falling apart" despite medical care.

Anabolic steroids have long been known to promote tissue growth and regeneration plus provide some pain relief. Arguably, these medicinals are underutilized in pain care and I believe they should be attempted in late stage, "falling apart" patients.

Unfortunately, since the 1984 Olympics, anabolic steroids have been condemned and almost regulated out of existence. Due to a need to assist the emerging debilitated group of chronic pain patients described above I have experimented with nandrolone. My experience is described below. My conclusion is that AS have a definite place in some late-stage, wasting, and/or deteriorating chronic pain patients.

In my long medical career, I have periodically been involved with anabolic steroids and have been part of their history in modern medicine. I have chosen to recap some of my experiences here as I believe they will bring some elucidation to an almost taboo subject.

My first encounter with anabolic steroids and pain is recalled in this vignette.

*It was late Fall of 1968. I was a new US Army Medical Officer. My first assignment after leaving residency and going active Army duty was taking care of soldiers in Brooke Army Hospital in San Antonio who had an infectious disease and were air evaced in from Vietnam. My second job landed me in Aschaffenburg, West Germany, a beautiful rustic town on the Main River. Stationed there was a brigade of the famed 3rd Infantry (Marne Division) that helped conquer Hitler in World War II. I was officially the medical doctor in charge of a tank battalion (4th and 64th). On my second day after arrival, I was called to be introduced to the Brigade Commander who was a most popular, competent, and respected colonel. I well remember his admonishment, "Doc, what we do here is train and retrain. We must be able on a day's notice to ship out to the Russian border, the middle east, or Vietnam. Do one thing, "Keep my boys ready at all times." There was no better advice for an army doctor, then or now. In less than a week I had to put this goal to the test. Ready or not on a Monday morning, one of our soldiers who had spent the weekend off base (known as "on the economy"), drank too much German wine, got into a few brawls, and managed to get a couple of tattoos. He showed up in our dispensary looking beat up, down and out, and in pain from a few crushed ribs, bruised joints, and bleeding tattoos. He was far from "ready" to fight for his country. I was baffled as to what to do so I consulted a doc, Don Warren, who had been on base for a couple of years. He knew both the medical and command goals of the 3rd brigade. Don said, "No problem, we have a treatment for pain and injury that puts these guys back to work in about a day." Much to my surprise, the treatment was a weak opioid, propoxyphene (Darvon®) and an anabolic steroid (dianabol or other). This combination was given to the trooper, and sure enough, within 24 hours he was back, full throttle, on duty and ready. For the next four years I gave the combination of*

*Darvon and an anabolic steroid to literally a few dozen soldiers who had pain and injury due to any number of causes. If one tried this effective treatment today in the United States, the doctor would probably be arrested. But at one time, this forgotten, but effective treatment of an opioid and AS helped keep some soldiers stay "ready."*

Between the 1960s and 1984, anabolic steroids were considered legitimate, medical treatment. Dr. Kerr, mentioned in a previous chapter, had dedicated his practice, near to my own, in San Gabriel, California, to over 15 years and 4000 patients who were either body builders or team athletes in baseball, football, and basketball. He used steroids to help body builders achieve a muscular, "cut" look to win contests. Team athletes simply needed bulk, speed, fast healing, and pain relief. Dr. Kerr could mix and match all the available anabolic steroids to fit his patient needs. In those days, he was regarded as a master of the athletic trade, highly respected, and highly sought after. I prescribed AS liberally in my pain clinic between 1975 and 1984 for patients who had become debilitated or wasted. They provided good pain relief for these late-stage pain patients, and they minimized the use of opioids and benzodiazepines. I found that they produced muscular strength and energy so a person might not be forced to use a wheelchair or be bound to couch or bed. Persons with less than a year to live, perked up, and seemed much more accepting of their fate when they could receive an AS with their opioids and other medications.

The world submerged a valuable pain care hormone in 1984. At the 1984 Olympics the East German and Russian women overwhelmingly won several of the events. When asked by media as to their secret of success, they openly declared they had training camps for their women athletes and administered AS to them. The news and media accounts caused such a fury after 1984 that AS have been essentially "missing in action." Anabolic steroids have been so "bad-mouthed," condemned and falsely accused of side effects since 1984 that doctors have almost stopped prescribing them. Today, they have been made controlled drugs like opioids, and doctors may be prosecuted if they regularly prescribe them. Between 1980 and 1984 I was a team doctor for the Los Angeles Dodgers. Like athletes everywhere, our players began to use them following the instructions laid down by Dr. Kerr. At that time, I didn't see medical harm of steroids among the athletes. They truly enhanced their athletic ability by strengthening muscles, nerves and other body tissues. This ability is not only wanted in sports, but it is obviously beneficial to a chronic pain patient.

I relate here a story that captures a lot of the societal rejection and emotions over AS in sports. In 1986 I was appointed as the Drug Advisor to the National Football League. My main job was to set up testing and treatment for players with drug (i.e., cocaine, marijuana) and/or alcohol dependency. Also, I was to assist team physicians find alternatives where possible to opioid use for injuries. My main contact was with each of 28 team doctors. For over 3 years the testing and treatment for abusable substances went well, and I personally enjoyed close contact with the commissioner (Pete Rozelle), coaches, owners, players, and doctors. By the late 1980s, however, the league was being pressured by all sorts of parties in and out of the NFL to ban AS. The major complaint was "the playing field needs to be level and equal" for everybody. AS provided too much advantage. I personally had reservations about the ban, but I was the drug advisor and took orders from the commissioner. I established an anabolic steroid testing program for the NFL by using the Olympic testing labs in Calgary, Tennessee, and UCLA. I also brought on some testing consultants. Our first session of testing players showed that about a third had an anabolic steroid in their urine. About that time attitudes about the AS ban changed. The league and the team doctors who sought the anabolic steroid ban began to wish they had never advocated for a test and ban program. The identification of star players caused chaos and disruption to the game. As head of the testing program, I personally became about as unpopular as a fox in a hen house. No one answered calls or wanted to meet for lunch. A key point here, however, is that I heard repeatedly from the team doctors that anabolic steroids did enhance athletic performance, but they also rapidly healed injuries and reduced pain.

Due to my involvement with anabolic steroids in the NFL, I became well-known in the sub-culture of anabolic steroid users. A few non-NFL athletes became addicted to them and voluntarily sought my care. I always maintained my own addiction and pain practice along with my part-time work in the professional sports world. I found a way to withdraw guys from steroids, and I also determined the scientific reason that anabolic steroids produced pain relief right along with healing and tissue generation. One of my cases was seminal, and I reported it in the New England Journal of Medicine (See references) with the title "Anabolic Steroid Dependence with Opioid-Type Features."

The case involved a 23-year-old body builder who was simultaneously using three different anabolic steroids (called "stacking"). After three years of use, he couldn't stop any one of them without experiencing withdrawal symptoms. I gave the young man injections of naloxone and caused a withdrawal reaction identical to that of opioid withdrawal. The classic opioid withdrawal symptoms include dilated pupils, sweating, hypertension, tachycardia, gooseflesh, and nausea. This finding proved one thing. AS have opioid properties and act by attaching to opioid receptors. The bottom line is this, AS simultaneously relieve pain and stimulate growth of body tissues. Also, like opioids, overuse can cause addiction with extended use.

Today's FDA label for anabolic steroids is basically for some testicular conditions and for "wasting conditions." Many chronic pain patients, particularly those with a connective tissue disease such as Ehlers-Danlos Syndrome, CRPS, or adhesive arachnoiditis (AA) or other "worst of the worst" painful condition reach a wasting or "falling apart" stage. They should have the benefits of an anabolic steroid.

Nandrolone is available for clinical use. It is available as a commercial injection, or it can be compounded as a capsule. Interestingly, it is produced as a trace hormone in the CNS, probably as a metabolite of DHEA. Its apparent natural use is that of neurogenic protection and healing.

To help determine nandrolone's role in chronic pain treatment, I and my research associate, Dr. Martin J. Porcelli, DO, conducted one open label trial. Nandrolone, in a dose of 25 to 50 mg twice a day, was given to 28 patients with intractable pain, adhesive arachnoiditis, and evidence of deterioration and wasting. Criteria for wasting included loss of muscle mass, weakness, and frail appearance. Patients were 18 men (64.2%) and 10 women (35.8%). All took opioid drugs and a variety of ancillary medications mainly neuropathic agents and anti-inflammatories. After 12 months an evaluation was done. All 28 reported that pain relief had improved. Patients all reported an increase in strength, energy, and mobility. Clinically they appeared less frail. Opioid reduction in the group was approximately 10-20%. No patient stopped opioids or became pain free. No patient, however, had worse symptomatology to include lower extremity paralysis or urinary/bowel incontinence. All patients desired to continue nandrolone. This study appeared to show that nandrolone improved pain control and slowed or stopped continued deterioration and wasting. It did not appear to have a dramatic effect on opioid reduction or reversal of the symptoms of adhesive arachnoiditis. Our conclusion is that nandrolone and other anabolic steroids should be given a trial in chronic pain patients who have reached a state of debilitation and wasting.

It can arguably be said that anabolic steroids are the most underutilized hormones in chronic pain treatment. The bias and negativity surrounding anabolic steroids in sports should not hold back their use in chronic pain treatment.

In summary, there is a growing group of severe chronic pain patients due to multiple causes that are ending up in a debilitated, deteriorating state. Anabolic steroids have a definite place in the treatment of those individuals.

TABLE

Quick Clinical Guide Nandrolone Administration

- 25 to 50 mg a day of compounded nandrolone for late-stage palliative pain patients who show evidence of wasting and debilitation

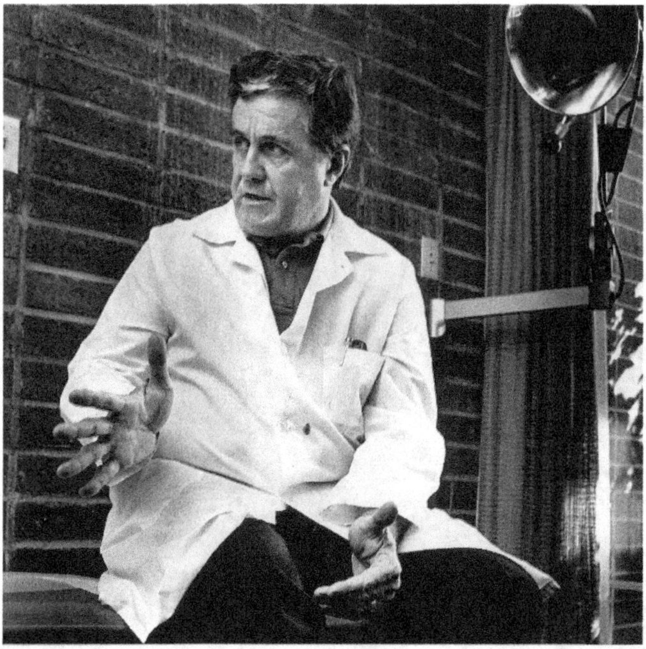

Dr. Robert Kerr openly prescribed steroids to about 4000 athletes including Olympic competitors from 19 countries as well as professional football, basketball, and baseball players. His book, now an "underground bible", explains how anabolic steroids provide athletic superiority plus healing and pain relief.

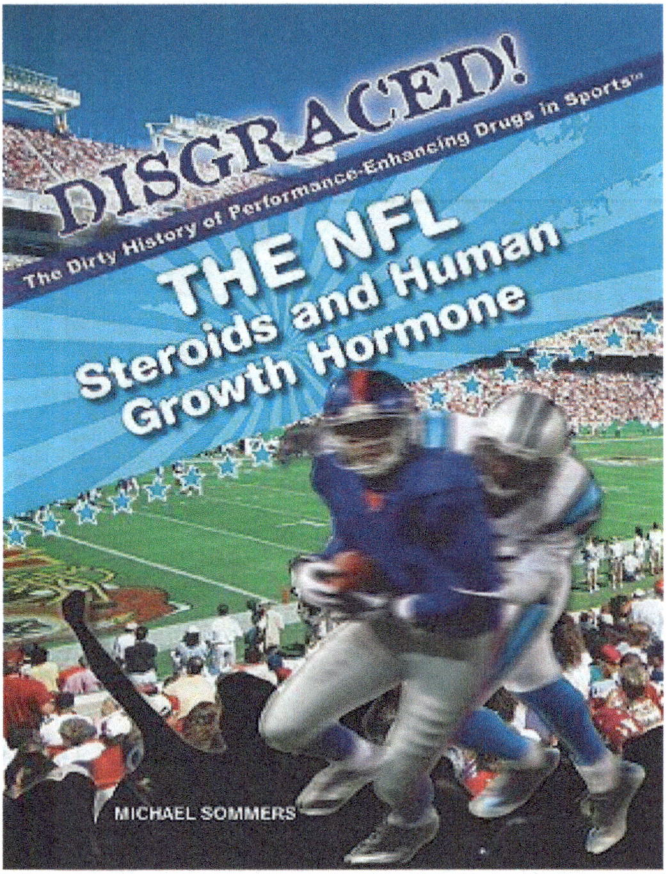


Headlines such as these examples compelled the National Football League to initiate anabolic steroid testing.

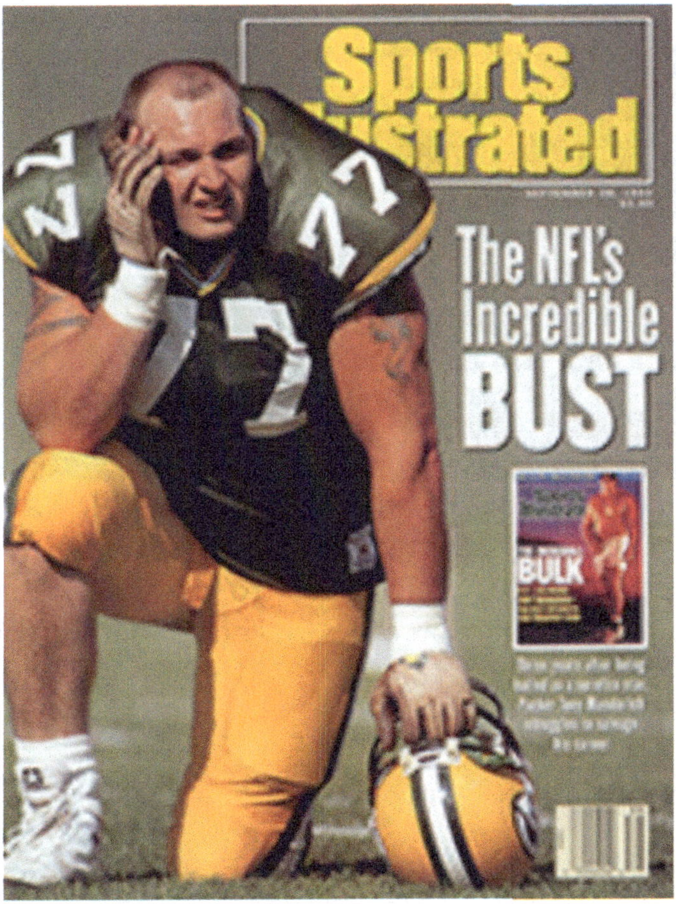
Sports
The NFL's
Incredible
BUST
BULK

1984 Olympian on Steroids – Silver Metal

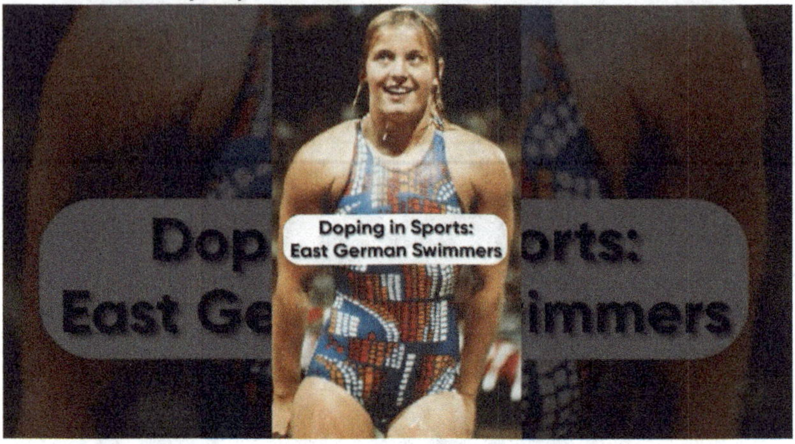


Pictorial example of an Olympic medal winner in 1984. Widespread media pictures such as this one enraged society which led to condemnation of anabolic steroids not only in sports but in medical practice.

## References

1. Aloisi AM, Ceccarelli I, Fiorenzani P, et al. Testosterone affects pain-related responses differently in male and female rats. Neurosci Lett 2004;361:262-264.
2. Fednekar J and Mulgacnker V. Role of testosterone on pain threshold in rats. *Indian J Physci Pharmacol* 1995;39:423-24.
3. Gascon A, Belvis JJ, Berisa F, et al. Nandrolone decanoate is a good alternative for the treatment of anemia in elderly male patients on hemodialysis. *Geriatr Nephrol Urol* 1999;9(2):67-72
4. Gold J, High HA, Li Y, et al. Safety and efficacy of nandrolone decanoate for treatment of wasting in patients with HIV infection. *AIDS* 1996 Jun;10(7):745-52.
5. Hamdy RC, Moore SW, Whalen KE, et al. Nandrolone decanoate for men with osteoporosis. *Amer J Ther* 1998 Mar;5(2):89-95.
6. Hassager C, Jensen LT, Podenphant J, et al. Collagen synthesis in post-menopausal women during therapy with anabolic steroid or female sex hormones. *Metabolism* 1990 Nov;39(11):1167-9.
7. Hau M, Dominguez OA, Evrard HC. Testosterone reduces responsiveness to nociceptive stimuli in a wild bird. *Horm Behav* 2004;46:165-170.
8. Jones KJ. Gonadal steroids and neuronal regeneration: a therapeutic role. *Adv Neurol* 1993;59:227-240.

9. Sattler FR, Jaque SV, Schroeder ET, et al. Effects of pharmacological doses of nandrolone decanoate and progressive resistance training in immunodeficient patients infected with human immunodeficiency virus. *J Clin Endocrinol Metab* 1999 Apr;84(4):1268-76.
10. Strawford A, Barbieri T, Neese R, et al. Effects of nandrolone decanoate therapy in borderline hypogonadal men with HIV-associated weight loss. *J Acquir Immune Defic Syndr Hum Retrovirol* 1999 Feb 1;20(2):137-46.
11. Tennant F, Black DL, Voy PO. Anabolic steroid dependence with opioid-type features. *N Eng J Med* 1988;319:578.

# 12. COLOSTRUM AND DEER ANTLER VELVET: MULTI-HORMONE FORMULATIONS

There are 2 hormonal preparations that contain multiple hormones plus a number of other autoimmune, anti-inflammatory, and regenerative medicinals. One is colostrum and the other is deer antler velvet. These two multi-hormonal preparations are becoming popular among chronic pain patients. Colostrum is secreted in breast milk by mammals for a few hours after they give birth. Its multiplicity of hormones and anti-infective agents are to protect the newborn and energize his/her metabolic systems that sustain life.

Antlers of some deer species contain a velvety tissue that has similar functions of a pituitary gland. This velvety substance has historically been a highly sought after medicinal. It once carried the name of "kings medicine."

Given the popular emergence of these two multi-hormonal therapies, some detail is presented here. Several years ago, the author first encountered colostrum in a woman with Ehlers-Danlos Syndrome (EDS) who had multiple painful conditions. She has lived into her 70's without the severe debilitation so common to persons with EDS. She attributes a lot of her success to colostrum which she has taken for 3 decades. Since then, I have reviewed many patients, especially those with EDS, who report positive effects with colostrum.

## Deer Antler Velvet

Deer antler velvet refers to the entire antler in its growth phase. It has been used in Chinese medicine for at least 2000 years and has recently re-emerged as a popular hormonal therapy. The chemical composition of deer antler velvet is highly complex containing 40 key compounds and 400 active ingredients. Pertinent to chronic pain care, deer antler velvet contains multiple hormones including several growth factors (See Table). Over the centuries it has been used to treat several dozen different medical conditions.

Deer antler velvet is marketed as a dietary supplement to support these conditions:

- Immune system
- Circulation and healing
- Sports nutrition and recovery
- Joint health and mobility

The recommended supplementary dose is 500 mg once or twice a day. Dosages above supplementary may range up to 3000 mg a day. At these high dosages it has been found to enhance athletic performance and some athletic organizations ban its use. It tends to build tissue and promote faster recovery and healing from injured tissues. It is Asian athletes who have primarily used deer antler velvet for athletic enhancement, but it is now commonly used by athletes in other countries.

## Colostrum

Colostrum is in the first milk that a mammal produces after pregnancy. This secretion of colostrum does not last for long; rather, it is created for the newborn to give it vital nutrients, antibodies, and other factors it needs right after birth. Therefore, after a few short days the production of colostrum all but stops.

Colostrum has been medicinally used for hundreds of years and over 1,000 clinical reports have been written about its use. To date, colostrum has been used and demonstrated to be safe for a variety of clinical conditions. These include viral illnesses, allergies and autoimmune diseases, heart disease, cancer, weight-loss programs, athletic stress, leaky gut syndrome, wound healing, and muscle repair and growth. In short, the most important components of colostrum can basically be broken down into two major categories: immunity modulator and hormonal growth factors. The major hormones in colostrum are listed in the Table. Colostrum is marketed as a dietary supplement in a dosage of about 1000 to

2000 mg per day. No systematic reports at higher dose usage are known to this author and no serious side effects are known.

## Best Use of Colostrum and Deer Antler Velvet

Should medical practitioners recommend colostrum or deer antler velvet to chronic pain patients? These two hormonal substances are similar to a multivitamin-mineral preparation. There may be no specific attribute, but they may provide generalized protective and regenerative action. Their use in chronic pain patients is relatively new. Reports to this author have included better pain control, greater strength, increased energy and mobility. No side effects are known at this time. It is entirely possible that dosages above supplementary use may provide potent anabolic and regenerative effects.

In the author's opinion the best use of these multi-component hormone preparations may be in patients who have multi-system pain conditions, genetic connective tissue diseases, or deteriorating or wasting states. Hopefully some of the many components in the compounds will slow or even halt degeneration and wasting.

<u>TABLE</u>

<u>Quick Clinical Guide</u>

Once a day supplement for multi-system pain patients, those in wasting or deterioration states and in genetic connective tissue diseases.

## TABLES

**Hormones in Colostrum**
Epidermal growth factor
Insulin-like growth factor
Transforming growth factor
Fibroblast growth factor
Platelet derived growth factor

**Hormones in Deer Antler Velvet**
Human growth hormone
Insulin-like growth factor
Transforming growth factor
Epidermal growth factor
Neurotrophins

## References


1. Buckley JD, Brinkworth GD, Abbot MJ. Effect of bovine colostrum on anaerobic exercise performance and plasma insulin-like growth factor I. *J Sports Sci* 2003;21:577-588.
2. Ko KM, Yip TT, Tsao SW, et al. Epidermal growth factor from deer (Cervus elaphus) submaxillary gland and velvet antler. *Gen Compar Endocrin* 1986;63:431-440.
3. Kotsis Y, Mikelidi A, Aresti C, et al. A low dose 6-week bovine colostrum supplementation maintains performance and attenuates inflammatory indices following a Loughborough Intermittent Shuttle Test in soccer players. *Eur J Nutr* 2018;57:181-1195.
4. Panahi Y, Falahi G, Falahpour M, et al. Bovine colostrum in the management of nonorganic failure to thrive: a randomized clinical trial. *J Pediatr Gastrointerol Nutr* 2010;50:551-554.
5. Pessi T, Isolauri E, Sutas Y, et al. Suppression of T-cell activation by Lactobacillus rhamnosus GG-degraded bovine casein. *Int Immunopharmacol* 2001;1:211-218.
6. Playford RT, Weiser MJ. Bovine colostrum: its constituents and uses. *Nutrients* 2021;13:265-268.
7. Satyaraj E, Reynolds A, Pelker R, et al. Supplementation of diets with bovine colostrum influences immune function in dogs. *Br J Nutr* 2013;110:2216-2221.

8. Wang BX, Zhao XH, Qi SB, et al. Stimulating effect of deer antler extract on protein synthesis in senescence-accelerated mice in vivo. *Chem Pharma Bulletin* 1988;36:2593-2598.
9. Wang BX, Zhao XH, Qi SB, et al. Effects of repeated administration of deer antler extract on biochemical changes related to ageing in senescence accelerated mice. *Chem Pharma Bulletin* 1988;36:2587-2592.
10. Wang BX, Chen X, ZhangW. Influence of the active compounds isolated from pilose antler on syntesis of protein and RNA in mouse liver. *Acta Pharma Sinica* 1990;25:321-325.

# 13. OXYTOCIN

Oxytocin is the only hormone whose only known function is to provide pain relief. It surges at the time of delivery to provide pain relief to assist a woman through the birthing process.

Oxytocin is naturally produced at low levels in both males and females. All of its functions are unknown, but it likely has some ongoing neuroprotection and regeneration properties that are continually operative. It surges at the time of an injury or emergence of pain.

Oxytocin is a powerful pain reliever with opioid potency. Produced in the hypothalamus, oxytocin is released into the peripheral circulation via the posterior pituitary, as well as into the central nervous system, including spinal fluid. At times of stress or pain, surges of oxytocin are released into the peripheral nervous system as well. There are neuronal projections from the hypothalamus to receptors in the dorsal horn of the spinal cord that function to prevent pain signals from reaching the brain. Oxytocin receptors also are located at multiple sites in the brain and throughout the spinal cord.

Oxytocin is very safe for pain relief. It is useful as either a flare or secondary agent. Considering its potency and safety, it is underused for pain relief.

It has a favorable safety profile, and I know of no cases of abuse or addiction. I have prescribed it both as a maintenance pain relief agent and for pain flares in lieu of an opioid. My patients with chronic pain conditions have received instructions to take oxytocin two or three times a day. The potency of a single oxytocin dose is about the equivalent of 30 mg of oxycodone or morphine.

A single dosage of oxytocin ranges from 20 to 40 international units (IU). It can be given as liquid sublingual drops or made into a troche. It can also be administered by the nasal route. In a small study I used ketamine simultaneously with oxytocin. Within 15 minutes after an oxytocin dose, a dose of liquid ketamine at a dose of 17.5 to 25 mg was given. When used together the two provided excellent pain relief. The patients who received these two agents in combination were long-time chronic pain patients who had previously used opioids. All reported that an oxytocin-ketamine combination produced pain relief equivalent to opioids.

Oxytocin is underutilized but is an excellent opioid alternative. It should be especially considered in patients who cannot obtain enough opioids for satisfactory pain relief.

TABLE

Quick Clinical Guide to Oxytocin Administration

- Give 20 to 40 units as a sublingual or buccal formulation for either pain relief or breakthrough/flare pain

## References

1. Breton JD, Veinante P, Uhl-Bronner S, et al. Oxytocin-induced antinociception in the spinal cord is mediated by a subpopulation of glutamatergic neurons in lamina I-II which amplify GABAergic inhibition. *Mol Pain* 2008;4:19.
2. Evans JJ. Oxytocin in the human-regulation of derivations and destinations. *Eur J Endocrinol*. 1997 Dec;137(6):559-71.
3. Gimpi G, Fahranholz F. The oxytocin receptor system: structure, function, and regulation. *Physiol Rev* 2001;81:629-683.
4. Goodin BR, Ness TJ, Robbins MT. Oxytocin-A multifunctional analgesic for chronic deep tissue pain. *Curr Pharm Res* 2015;21:906-913.
5. Goodin BR, Ness TJ, Robbins MT. Oxytocin-A multifunctional analgesic for chronic deep tissue pain. *Curr Pharm Res* 2015;21:906-913.
6. Paloyels Y, Krahe C, Maltegos S, et al. The analgesic effect of oxytocin in humans: a double-blind placebo controlled cross-over study using laser-evoked potentials. *J Neuroendocrin* 2015;Doi:10:1111.
7. Rash JA, Aguirre-Camacho A, Campbell TS. Oxytocin and pain: a systemic review and synthesis of findings. *Clin J Pain* 2014;30:453-462.
8. Rash JA, Campbell TS. The effect of intranasal oxytocin administration on acute cold pressor pain: a placebo-controlled, double-blind,

within-subjects crossover trial. *Psychosom Med* 2014;76(6):422-429.
9. Rook JA, Aguirre-Camacho A, Campbell TS. Oxytocin and pain: a systematic review and synthesis of findings. *Clin J Pain* 2013;00:1-9.
10. Stock S, Uvnus-Moberg K. Increased plasma levels of oxytocin in response to afferent electrical stimulation of the sciatic and vaga acrves and in response to touch and pinch in anaesthetized rats. *Acta Physiol Scand* 1988;132:29-34.
11. Tennant F. Oxytocin in intractable pain patient unresponsive to standard treatments. *Amer Pain Soc*, Tampa, 2014.
12. Tennant F, Pedersen C. Sublingual oxytocin and ketamine for pain relief. *Pain Week*, Las Vegas, 2017.
13. Tennant F. Combined use of oxytocin and human chorionic gonadotropin in intractable pain patients. *Pain Med* 2014;15(3):519.
14. Wong YL, Yuan Y, Yang J, et al. The interaction between the oxytocin and pain modulation in headache patients. *Neuropeptides* 2003;97:93-97.
15. Yang J. Intrathecal administration of oxytocin induces analgesia in low back pain involving the endogenous opiate peptide system. *Spine* 1994;19:867-871.
16. Yang J, Yang Y, Chen JM, et al. Central oxytocin enhances antinociception in the rat. *Peptides* 2007;28:1113-1119.

# 14. PRICED OUT OF USE: HUMAN GROWTH HORMONE (HGH) AND ANDRENOCORTICOTROPIN (ACTH)

In earlier chapters I wrote about the tragic, scandalous, deceitful events that led to the deprivation of estrogen and anabolic steroids for chronic pain patients. Unfortunately, human growth hormone (HGH) and adrenocorticotropin (ACTH) are essentially not available for pain care, because they are too expensive. Based on my experience and study of these two hormones, like estrogen and anabolic steroids, they should be available for pain practitioners to prescribe to any chronic pain patient. Many would undoubtedly benefit from them.

First, why aren't HGH and ACTH being used? This appears to simply be a matter of cost and bias. Both compounds cost thousands of dollars a month. Insurance companies only pay this ultra-high dollar cost for some very specific diseases. Chronic pain isn't one of these. In the past before cost became a barrier, I made good use of both hormones in select chronic pain patients. There are other positive reports. Dr. Bennett of the University of Oregon found HGH to be particularly effective in the treatment of fibromyalgia. In years past I had been able to secure HGH for some patients with Ehlers-Danlos Syndrome (EDS). I believe the results were most positive, and I argue that every person with EDS should have a trial with HGH.

Adrenocorticotropin (ACTH) is the hormone produced in the pituitary that stimulates the adrenals and gonads to produce cortisol and other hormones. Prior to this century, ACTH (trade name Acthar®) was inexpensive and readily available for clinical use by all medical practitioners. A single dose used to cost pennies. Consequently, in the 1980s and 90s this author gave 1cc injections routinely when patients attended his pain clinic for their monthly visit. The injection was praised by patients because it improved pain relief, energy, and motivation. Patients voluntarily asked for it and were not forced to take it. Unfortunately, ACTH is now only marketed by a single company for special monopolistic sales. Now it is very expensive and beyond the ability of routine pain care to afford it.

References

1. Bagge E, Bengtsson B, Carisson L, Et al. Low growth hormone secretion in patients with fibromyalgia-a preliminary report on 10 patients and 10 controls. *J of Rheum* 1998;25:146-148.
2. Balva ES, Deodhar A, Jones KD, et al. Impaired growth hormone secretion in fibromyalgia patients. *Arth and Rheum* 2002;46:1344-1350.
3. Bennett R, Clark S, Campbell S, et al. Low levels of somatomedin-C in patients with fibromyalgia. *Arthritis Rheum* 1992;35:1113-1116.
4. Bennett RM, Clark SR, Burkhardt CS, et al. A randomized double-blind placebo-controlled study of growth hormone in the treatment of fibromyalgia. *Amer J of Med* 1998;04:227-231.

# 15. HORMONES AND PEPTIDES

This book would not be complete without mentioning the very recent combined use of hormones and peptides. Polypeptides are chains of two or more amino acids. Some very innovative and creative entrepreneurs have put together chains of amino acids that, in typical peptide fashion, enter specific biologic, metabolic pathways to produce a therapeutic effect. Most of the available peptides have been created to regenerate or regrow damaged or diseased tissues.

Some peptides have autoimmune, anti-inflammatory properties (i.e., thymosin) and antioxidant activity (i.e., glutathione). A few peptides have already become popular with severe chronic pain patients (See Table). When combined with a hormone that has regeneration or regrowth properties, (i.e., HCG, DHEA, nandrolone) there clinically appears to be great synergism. Although no systematic data on effectiveness is yet available, I am personally receiving reports from patients who are reducing their pain and disease impairments by the combined use of a regenerative hormone and a peptide. Some examples of the combined use are DHEA and BPC-157, and HCG and ARA 290. Although the combined use of hormones and peptides is too early to make recommendations and proclamations, early experience and anecdotal reports suggest that this measure is a significant advance in chronic pain care.

TABLE

Popular Peptides in Chronic Pain Care

- ✓ KPV – lysine, proline, valine
- ✓ Body protection compound – BPC-157
- ✓ Thymosin
- ✓ Glutathione
- ✓ ARA 290 – cibinetide

## Summary

Enough knowledge and experience have now accumulated on hormonal therapies to incorporate them into modern chronic pain care. Some hormones heal and regenerate damaged or injured tissue responsible for a chronic pain condition and others enhance opioids and other medicinals for pain relief.

Modern day chronic pain treatment provides a wide array of pharmacologic, physical, and surgical measures that have benefitted millions of persons throughout the world. Hormonal therapies enhance pain care and can be added to current pain treatment measures.

# Index

<u>OTHER BOOKS BY FOREST TENNANT</u>

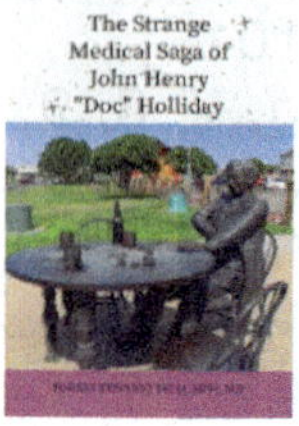


The Strange Medical Saga of "John Henry

ISBN: 9781955934275
LOC: 2023913628

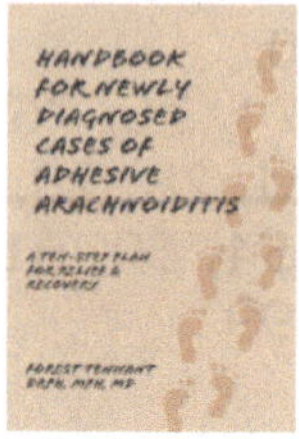


Handbook For Newly Diagnosed Cases of Adhesive Arachnoiditis

ISBN: 9781955934244
LOC: 2023908116

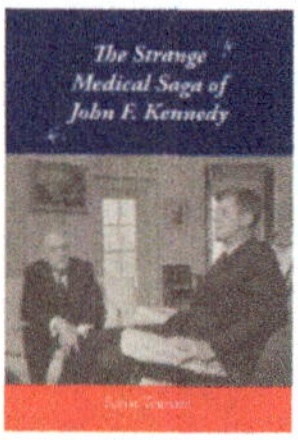


The Strange Medical Saga of JFK

ISBN: 9781955934213
LOC: 2023903440

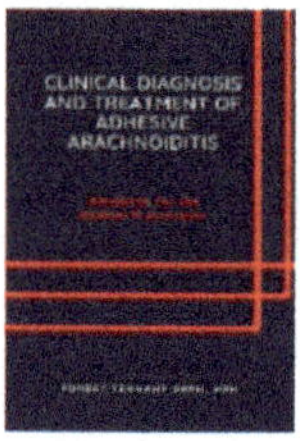


Clinical Diagnosis and Treatment of Adhesive Arachnoiditis

ISBN: 9781955934183
LOC: 2022907190

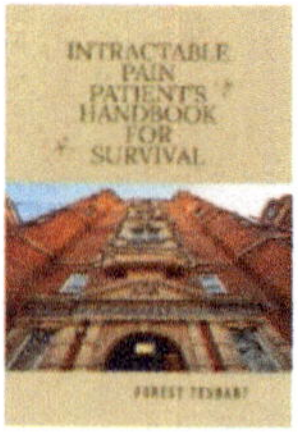


Intractable Pain Patients Handbook for Survival

ISBN: 9781955934121
LOC: 2021916464

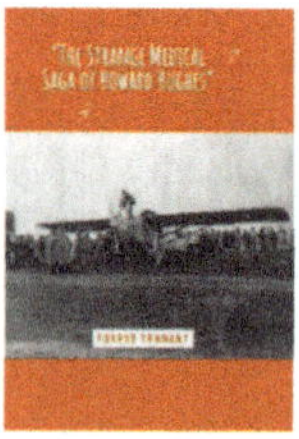

The Strange Medical Saga of Howard Hughes

ISBN: 9781955934091
LOC: 2021912855

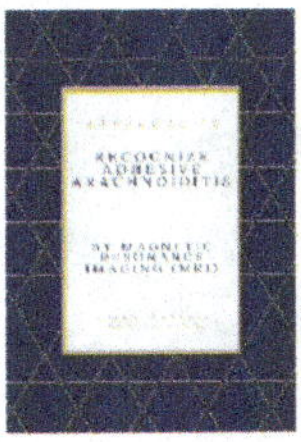

Handbook To Recognize Adhesive Arachnoiditis by Magnetic Resonance Imaging (MRI)

ISBN: 9781955934152
LOC: 2021925161

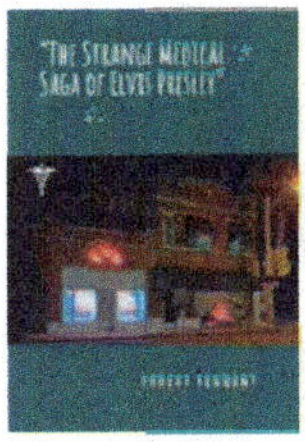

The Strange Medical Saga of Elvis

ISBN: 9781955934008
LOC: 2021911718

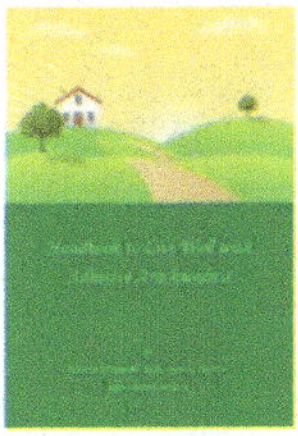

Handbook to Live Well with Adhesive Arachnoiditis

ISBN: 978195934060
LOC: 2021912718

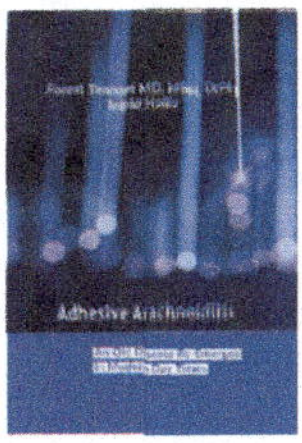

An Old Disease Re-Emerges in Modern Times

ISBN: 9781955934039
LOC: 2021912467

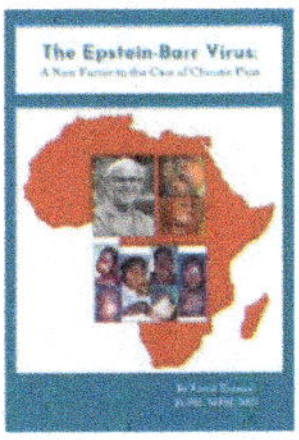

The Epstein-Barr Virus: A New Factor in the Care of Chronic Pain

ISBN: 9781955934428
LOC: 2024919179

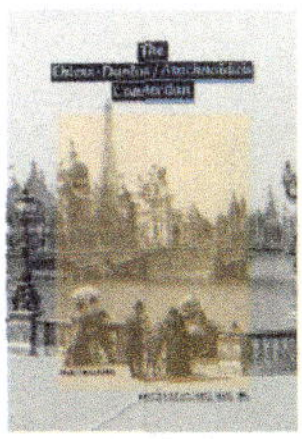

The Ehlers-Danlos / Arachnoiditis Connection

ISBN: 9781955934381
LOC: 2024911409

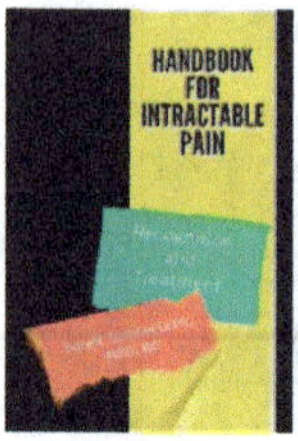


Handbook for Intractable Pain

ISBN: 9781955934329
LOC: 2023921074

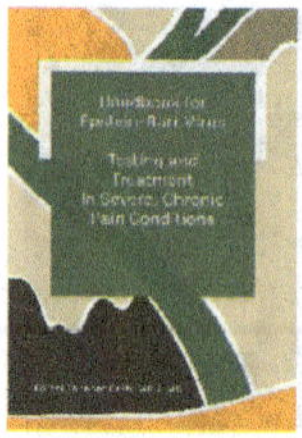


Handbook for Epstein-Barr Virus

ISBN: 9781955934459
LOC: 20249226413

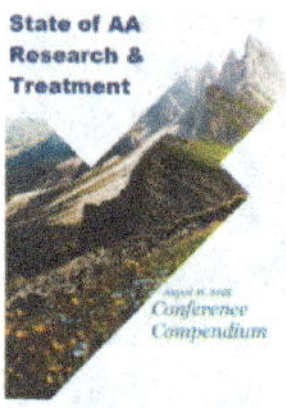


State of AA Research & Treatment Conference 2025

ISBN: 9781955934503
LOC: 2025918282

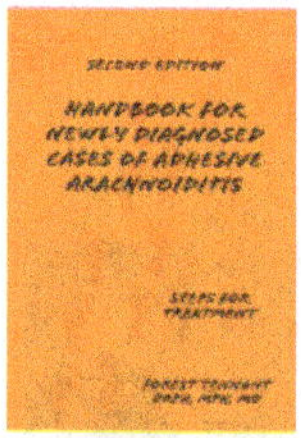


Second Edition Handbook For Newly Diagnosed Cases of Adhesive Arachnoiditis

ISBN: 9781955934480
LOC: 2025912299

Made in United States
North Haven, CT
01 March 2026

89296299R00068